Get Through

Postgraduate Medical Interviews

Kaji Sritharan MBBS BSc MRCS (Eng)

Specialist Registrar in General Surgery, Northwest Thames Rotation,
London & Honorary Clinical Research Fellow, Division of Surgery, Oncology,
Reproductive Biology and Anaesthetics, Imperial College London

Nigel Standfield MBBS FRCS FRCS (Ed.)

Head of the London School of Surgical Specialties, London Deanery; and
Consultant Vascular Surgeon & Honorary Clinical Senior Lecturer,
Imperial Academic Health Sciences Centre, London

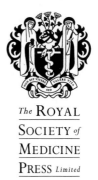

The ROYAL
SOCIETY of
MEDICINE
PRESS Limited

British Library Cataloguing in Publication Data
A catalogue record for this book is available from the British Library

ISBN: 978-1-85315-816-2

Distribution in Europe and Rest of the World:
Marston Book Services Ltd
PO Box 269
Abingdon
Oxon OX14 4YN, UK
Tel: +44 (0)1235 465500
Fax: +44 (0)1235 465555
Email: direct.order@marston.co.uk

Distribution in USA and Canada:
Royal Society of Medicine Press Ltd
c/o BookMasters Inc
30 Amberwood Parkway
Ashland, OH 44805, USA
Tel: +1 800 247 6553/ +1 800 266 5564
Fax: +1 410 281 6883
Email: order@bookmasters.com

Distribution in Australia and New Zealand:
Elsevier Australia
30–52 Smidmore Street
Marrickville NSW 2204, Australia
Tel: +61 2 9517 8999
Fax: +61 2 9517 2249
Email: service@elsevier.com.au

Typeset by Phoenix Photosetting, Chatham, Kent
Printed in the UK by Bell & Bain Ltd, Glasgow

Contents

Preface

Following short-listing, the interview is the final and toughest hurdle standing between a candidate and their career path of choice. For most there will only be one chance and competition, especially in the wake of Modernising Medical Careers (MMC), has never been fiercer.

Get Through Postgraduate Medical Interviews aims to forearm candidates with the most up-to-date practical advice on how to maximize their chances of success in the postgraduate medical interview. Written in a format that lends itself to easy reading and information access, this book systematically and logically examines the entire interview process from start to finish; dispelling common myths and advising candidates on how to prepare, what to expect and what will be expected of them. In addition, it gives guidance on approaching commonly encountered 'hot interview topics' and on tackling those 'awkward' interview questions. *Get Through Postgraduate Medical Interviews* also offers advice on constructing a portfolio and tips on how to sell your best attributes and maximize your chances of success on the day.

Kaji Sritharan
Nigel Standfield

1 Introduction

The purpose of the interview

The interview is often the final and greatest obstacle between you and your chosen career. This is your opportunity to demonstrate that, not only are you the person you say you are on your application form, but that you are the best person for the job.

The interview should be approached as you would any exam or viva and the key to maximizing your chances of success on the day is thorough and meticulous preparation.

It is important to note that this book is simply an aid to the interview and, although the information within this book was accurate at the time of writing, with Modernising Medical Careers (MMC) still in its infancy, the selection and interview processes are still evolving, and the MMC website should be consulted for the most up-to-date information regarding the selection and interview process.

Arguably, why write this book now? With competition for posts never greater than at present, if you are lucky to be shortlisted for interview, your performance on the day will be instrumental to your success. The aim of this book is to equip you with the essential skills to tackle the interview and the variations that you could encounter, and to give you a better understanding of the interview process as a whole, putting you ahead of the game.

What is MMC?

The process to streamline training in the UK was initiated following publication of a document entitled *Unfinished Business*: *Proposals for Reform of the Senior House Officer Grade* (DH 2002), which recognized that there was a 'bottleneck' at senior house officer (SHO) level and that a large number of SHOs – a so-called 'lost tribe' – would never progress through to higher specialist training. It was felt that this was a waste of talent and that trainees should be directed into a clear training pathway at an earlier stage of their training. MMC is based upon the principle of having a defined competency-based (not time-based) curriculum for postgraduate training, with broad-based, flexible training in the early stages (the Foundation programme), followed by seamless progression through speciality training.

The principles of MMC are commendable and should not be confused with the Medical Training Application Service (MTAS) – the centralized electronic portal devised for national recruitment and selection of junior doctors into speciality training posts, which in 2007 failed causing a fiasco that should not be repeated.

The application process

Due to the collapse of MTAS in 2007, there will be *no* national computer-based system for applications to speciality training posts in 2008, and the majority of interviews will be conducted at a deanery level.

Plans for recruitment in 2009 are still under discussion following the Tooke Report (an independent review conducted by Sir John Tooke into Modernising Medical Careers [MMC]).

Recruitment in 2008

Recruitment into speciality training in 2008 will be determined locally by individual deaneries, as pre-MTAS (except in a few specialities, namely, cardiothoracic surgery, paediatric surgery, plastic surgery and histopathology, where national selection has been agreed), and will be staggered, with deaneries advertising vacancies (these should include details ± job descriptions of the speciality training as well as fixed term speciality training appointments available), shortlisting candidates for interview using their own criteria and scoring systems, conducting interviews, selecting candidates and making job offers.

There will no longer be a single entry as in 2007, but deaneries and specialities will decide the entry dates. There will, however, be no more than three recruitment processes each year, and August is likely to continue to be the main recruiting time point. The other recruitment exercises are likely to occur in June and September in 2008. Although each deanery will have its own application form, these are likely to take on the format of a structured curriculum vitae (CV) with speciality-specific questions.

Trainees will be allowed to apply to as many deaneries and as many specialities as they wish, and information regarding the availability of posts will be updated regularly on the MMC and on each deanery's websites, which you are strongly recommended to keep viewing at regular intervals. Jobs will be advertised for a minimum of 72 hours before the closure to new applications but, for round 1, it is likely the timeframe for applying will be significantly longer. It is, however, worthwhile submitting your application as early as possible (see *Box 1.1*).

Box 1.1   Deaneries in the UK

There are 18 deaneries in the UK. These include:
- Defence Postgraduate Medical Deanery
- East Midlands Healthcare
- East of England Multi-Professional Deanery
- Kent, Surrey and Sussex (KSS) Deanery
- Leicestershire, Northamptonshire and Rutland (LNR) Deanery
- London Deanery
- Mersey Deanery
- NHS West Midlands Workforce Deanery
- North Western Deanery
- Northern Deanery
- Northern Ireland Deanery
- Oxford Deanery
- Scottish deaneries: East, North, South-East and West
- Severn Deanery
- South West Peninsula Deanery
- South Yorkshire and South Humber (SYSH) Deanery
- Trent Deanery
- Wales Deanery
- Wessex Deanery
- Yorkshire Deanery.

Run-through training and the transition

In 2007, the majority of specialist training posts were offered on a 'run-through' basis and these posts will be honoured. Thus, providing as a 'run-through' trainee you progress adequately as determined at your Annual Review of Competence Progression (ARCP), you will be guaranteed seamless progression to your Certificate of Completion of Training (CCT).

Others in 2007 were given 1-year appointments known as fixed term speciality training appointments (FTSTAs). With the completion of round 2 in 2007, and many posts still unfilled, a process of appointing locum appointments for service (LASs) was put into place. These LAS posts were appointments of 1 year or less and ultimately became very similar to FTSTAs, although, unlike the latter, not all LASs were educationally approved posts.

In 2008, 'run-through' training will only be offered in certain specialities and in the remainder of ST1/ST2, newly termed 'core' training will be 'uncoupled' from higher speciality training (see *Table 1.1*). Following speciality core training (CT1, CT2 and CT3), there will then be open competition into ST3 or ST4 (much like under the old Calman system of training). Core training is a term that will apply to core medical training, the acute care common stem, core surgical training and core psychiatric training and, except in psychiatry, will be for 2 years (in psychiatry, core training will be for 3 years).

The number of posts available at each level will be determined by the MMC Programme Board, and you should visit the MMC and Deanery websites at regular intervals for this information.

TABLE 1.1 Summary of specialities that in 2008 will offer 'run-through training' and those in which core training will be 'uncoupled' from higher specialist training

Offer of run-through training in 2008	Offer with uncoupling in 2008
Chemical Pathology	Anaesthesia
Clinical Radiology	Cardiothoracic Surgery
General Practice	Emergency Medicine
Histopathology	General Medicine
Medical Microbiology	General Surgery
Neurosurgery	Occupational Medicine
Obstetrics and Gynaecology	Oral and Maxillofacial Surgery
Ophthalmology	Otolaryngology (ENT)
Paediatrics and Child Health	Paediatric Surgery
Public Health Medicine	Plastic Surgery
	Psychiatry
	Trauma and Orthopaedic Surgery
	Urology

Closed versus open interviews

There will almost certainly, in most deaneries, be a closed interview process for the matching of run-through applicants to the appropriate posts. The principle of a closed interview is that the trainee is interviewed by the interview panel but not in competition with anyone else for that number. If they are successful in that interview, then they will progress through higher speciality training. If they are unsuccessful in that interview, they will repeat the year and will then have a further closed interview. Those posts, which are not filled by run-through training groups (RTGs) in closed interviews, will be advertised for open interview – i.e., offered in open competition to anyone that fulfils the personal specifications.

National selection

Some specialities and some sub-specialities have decided that because they are small they will move towards national selection, e.g., cardiothoracic surgery. The principle of national selection is that all of the applicants for that speciality will be processed at a single deanery, which will be nominated as the deanery responsible for that national selection. All shortlisted candidates will then be interviewed at that deanery by representatives of the different training programmes throughout the UK, and those candidates selected at interview will be offered the available posts. The top-ranked candidate will almost certainly get their first-choice post, the second ranked will then be given their choice of post and so forth down the ranks. National selection can only really work for small specialities with a small number of posts available.

What are speciality schools?

Speciality schools are deanery structures for managing speciality training. They provide a structure for educational governance and each speciality school will have a board comprised of representatives from each of the relevant stakeholders. The board, through the head of school, will contribute to the delivery of training and be responsible for maintaining the level of excellence of the training delivered. The speciality schools are designed to work closely with the Royal Colleges and the deanery as well as other NHS providers of training (e.g. Trusts).

What is the National Recruitment Office for general practice training?

The National Recruitment Office coordinates the national assessment and selection process for general practice speciality training programmes, which is composed of essentially four stages:

- *Stage 1 – Longlisting*: This follows the application process and, provided the application meets the necessary essential eligibility criteria, the application will be passed through for shortlisting.
- *Stage 2 – Shortlisting*: The shortlisting process in general practice requires the trainee to attend an initial assessment, which is conducted under examination conditions. Stage 2 assessments are conducted in one day within deaneries across the UK.
- *Stage 3 – Selection*: Invitation to attend a selection centre depends upon the score obtained in the assessment at stage 2, as well as the geographical preference given and the availability of places. At the selection centre, candidates are requested to undertake a series of exercises that are observed by trained assessors. These often include a patient simulation exercise, a group exercise and a written exercise. It is to be noted that there are no interviews.
- *Stage 4 – Allocation and job offer*: Allocation of a job to successful candidates is dependent upon their performance at the selection centre, the training programme requirements and the availability of a suitable vacancy.

Assessing the competition

In 2007 in England, there were approximately 28,000 applicants competing for 15,500 training places – a ratio of approximately 2:1. In 2008, it is predicted that the competition will be fiercer, with an overall ratio of more than 3:1 applicants per place. This is the average number of applicants across all specialities and, naturally, the competition for training places will vary according to the speciality.

The latest information from the MMC Programme Board estimated there to be between 8900 and 9100 posts available in 2008. Of these, 6100 are for entry at ST1, 2070 for entry at ST2 and only between 750 and 950 for ST3 for the whole of 2008. The total number of ST3 posts advertised in the January to May recruitment period is thought to be approximately 550, with the remainder advertised later in the year.

Table 1.2 gives a summary of the approximate number of applicants for each

TABLE 1.2 Summary of the approximate number of applicants per speciality both overall and for each individual deanery following the first round of applications in 2007

Speciality	Applications per post														Overall
	East of England	LNR	London/ KSS	Mersey	Northern	North Western	Oxford	Severn	South West	SYSH	Trent	Wessex	West Midlands	Yorkshire	
Acute medicine	5.3	4.0	3.3		8.8	9.8	5.6	9.0	3.0	6.3		5.0	13.7	7.9	5.6
Allergy			1.0												1.0
Anaesthesia	10.3	5.9	4.6	7.3	8.8	10.3	10.2	8.5	7.7	6.3	6.7	8.2	12.4	10.1	7.0
Audiological medicine			2.0												2.0
Cardiology	18.3		11.6	26.5	17.1	17.9	36.0	16.2		10.0	9.0	19.3	22.8	21.2	15.0
Cardiothoracic surgery			36.5		54.0	63.0							74		53.2
Clinical genetics			4.7	1.0	3.0	5.0	9.0	3.0		2.0				2.5	3.9
Clinical neurophysiology			1.0	4.0	5.0			10.0							2.3
Clinical oncology	15.0		6.1	1.0						6.0	1.0	2.0	7.6	7.0	5.9
Clinical pharmacology and therapeutics			0.0												0.0
Dermatology	13.5	8.5	11.6	5.0	10.0	9.3	13.0	15.0	6.8	10.5	6.0	13.0	8.5	7.4	9.1
Emergency medicine	6.1	6.5	4.0	6.0	5.8	15.0	11.2	8.0	2.0	5.3	4.8		4.8		5.5
Endocrinology and diabetes	10.3	12.0	5.5	13.3	12.4		7.0		6.5		5.0		13.3	12.5	8.9
Gastroenterology	19.0		8.7	17.3	21.4			21.0				14.3	23.0		13.2
General practice	4.3	1.5	2.5	5.7	19.5	3.7	4.6	5.1		9.0		4.7	3.7		3.6
General surgery	35.0	13.6	12.7	13.1	27.9	25.9	25.3	23.0	15.7	16.3	17.3		32.2	29.4	20.3
Genito-urinary medicine	10.0		5.4	4.0	6.0	7.8	14	9.7		7.5	6.5	10.5	14.0	8.0	5.4
Geriatric medicine	10.3	5.5	4.7	6.0	12.0	22.0	17.5	13.5					8.2		5.3
Haematology	5.0	8.0	4.5						5.0			13.0	11.6		6.8
Immunology		1.0	1.0			0.0	0.0								0.6
Infectious diseases	9.0	1.0	7.8			18.0	15.5			9.0	1.0		13.0		9.1
Infectious diseases and MMV – Medical microbiology	5.0		4.3								1.0			3.0	4.2
Infectious diseases and MMV – Virology			6.0							1.0					3.5
Medical oncology			6.0	4.0		8.7				10.0	10.0		7.6	13.0	7.1
Medical ophthalmology															1.5*
Neurology	2.0		11.3	11.0	14.7	12.7	32.7	58.0		10.0		18.0	10.5	26.0	14.4
Neurosurgery		12.5	6.3		5.5	2.0		23.0					1.0	19.0	10.2
Nuclear medicine			1.0												1.0
Obstetrics and gynaecology	17.7		5.6	9.5	11.5	16.2	17.8	8.2	10.0	10.1	15.5		19.7	12.2	9.4
Occupational medicine			4.0		3.0		3.0						2.0	4.0	3.0
Ophthalmology	19.0	13.0	5.5	12.9	8.5	14.0	22.0	9.0	9.0	13.0	12.0	15.0	20.7	16.7	10.8
Otolaryngology (ENT)	32.0		14.1		17.0	22.6			17.7	19.0	13.0	21.5	33.3	24.7	19.8
Paediatric surgery		36.0	9.7	23.0	6.2	15.0							32.0		15.9
Paediatrics	8.6	8.4	4.3	7.3	17.5	11.1	12.0	7.2	3.3	7.2	4.0	5.6	10.4	11.3	6.6
Palliative medicine	29.0		8.6		18.1	22.0	18.3					20.0	19.0	24.0	12.2
Plastic surgery			18.9	13.5	5.3	18.8	20.5		19.3	6.5	12.0		18.0	20.1	18.1
Psychiatry	11.4	8.5	3.6	6.3	1.0	8.4	14.4	6.6	3.5	6.0	4.0	10.9	9.1	7.7	6.1
Rehabilitation medicine	1.0		4.0	2.0	10.8	3.5	1.0	2.0	2.3		4.0	1.5	2.8	1.7	1.9
Renal medicine	8.7	3.0	7.0	5.5	13.1	11.5		10.0		6.0	5.0	5.0	13.8	9.0	7.7
Respiratory medicine	15.3	15.0	6.2	10.8	9.0	18.5	7.5						14.4	13.5	10.3
Rheumatology	5.0		12.3			16.0	23.7	10.5	4.5	13.0			8.3	9.8	7.8
Sports and exercise medicine			9.3		22.0										11.8
Trauma and orthopaedic surgery	28.5	20.3	14.6	24.3	29.4	33.4		23.3		30.0			35.9	28.2	22.6
Urology	33.0	15.0	8.5	23.0	25.3	31.0	24.0	23.3	30.0	14.3	14.3	40.0	37.0	25.0	17.6

*Average overall data; data from individual deaneries not available.

KSS, Kent, Surrey and Sussex; LNR, Leicestershire, Northamptonshire & Rutland; MMV, Medicines for Malaria Venture; SYSH, South Yorkshire and South Humber.

speciality and (with the exception of the Northern Ireland, Welsh and Scottish deaneries) for each individual deanery, as well as the average number of applicants for each speciality in the UK in the first round of applications in 2007.

In addition, it is useful to note that after the round 1 applications in 2007, shortages for applicants still existed in the following specialities:

- Anaesthetics
- Obstetrics and Gynaecology
- Paediatrics
- Psychiatry
- Geriatric Medicine.

The application ratios listed below, although useful guides to the level of competition within a speciality, should by no means be the sole factor influencing your career choice. Competition ratios will vary from year to year – those last year may not necessarily reflect the competition this year – and competition can be difficult to predict accurately, especially in margin specialities such as ENT or audiology.

The strength of competition will inevitably affect the likelihood of you being successfully selected into popular specialities, such as cardiothoracic surgery, general surgery and cardiology, and if your application is weak you may want to consider applying for more than one speciality. In these 'high-competition' specialities it is worthwhile seeking honest advice as to your realistic chance of succeeding, given your experience and credentials. Independent advice can be sought from:

- The appropriate Royal College
- Your clinical tutor or educational supervisor
- A deanery advisor.

Overseas graduates

Following the case brought by the British Association of Physicians of Indian Origin (BAPIO) against the Department of Health in 2007, and the Court of Appeal ruling in favour of BAPIO, applications by international medical graduates to speciality training posts cannot and will no longer be restricted.

Academic clinical fellowships

The recruitment process for academic clinical fellowships (ACFs) was launched by the National Institute for Health Research Capacity Development Programme, with the application process managed jointly by deaneries and universities.

Approximately 250 fellowships will be available in 2008. Doctors and dentists entering speciality training, including those with a national training number, are eligible to apply, and this does *not* exclude applying for non-academic speciality training posts.

Academic Clinical Fellows will have 25% of their time protected for academic activities, and need to be able to demonstrate 'outstanding potential for development as a clinical academic in research and/or education' in order to be considered for shortlisting.

Deferred entry

If you are already enrolled in a higher degree (e.g., MD or PhD) programme you should still apply but defer your start date. This can be for up to 3 years from the start of the course. If you wish to defer you should indicate this intent on your application form.

Flexible training

Theoretically at least, it should be easier to train flexibly under MMC due to the move away from time-served training to competency-based training, and the establishment of clearly defined competencies. If you are considering training flexibly then you should contact the deanery or your speciality school of training, and it is advisable to do this after the interview process. If you are eligible for flexible training and each case is considered individually, then you will need to apply to the deanery's Flexible Training Office for approval as well as funding. Under flexible training, you are required to work a minimum of 50% and a maximum of 90% of full-time hours.

Opportunities to train flexibly also exist at Foundation level; if interested, you should contact the deanery and aim to apply early.

Reference

Department of Health. (2002) *Unfinished Business: Proposals for Reform of the Senior House Officer Grade.* A report by Sir Liam Donaldson, Chief Medical Officer for England. DH, London. http://www.mmc.nhs.uk/Docs/Unfinished-Business.pdf

Useful links

MMC England: http://www.mmc.nhs.uk
MMC Scotland: http://www.mmc.scot.nhs.uk
MMC Wales: http://www.mmcwales.org
MMC Northern Ireland: http://www.nimdta.gov.uk/mmc
List of deanery websites: http://www.mmc.nhs.uk/default.aspx?page=284

2 Before the interview

Deciding level of entry into speciality training

Entry into the medical and surgical specialities is at three separate levels: ST1, ST2 and ST3. A person specification is published for each speciality (available on the MMC website), and the suitability for entry into each level is determined by the essential selection criteria. However, if you can tick all of the desirable boxes this will undoubtedly increase your chances of being shortlisted for interview.

Person specifications

The person specifications differ for each speciality but have a similar framework. The core criteria evaluated at ST3 include:

1. Qualifications

   - MBBS or equivalent (essential)

   - Postgraduate examinations, e.g., MRCP (essential)

2. Eligibility

   - Full GMC registration at the time of appointment (essential)

   - Evidence of achieving Foundation competencies in line with *Good Medical Practice* (GMC 2006) (essential)

   - Evidence of achieving ST1/ST2 competencies in speciality (essential)

   - Eligibility to work in the UK (essential)

3. Fitness to practice

4. Language skills

- Sufficient and demonstrable written and spoken skills in English (essential)

5. Health
   - Professional health standards in line with *Good Medical Practice* (GMC 2006) (essential)

6. Career progression
   - Ability to provide appointment history (essential)
   - At least 24 months' experience at senior house officer (SHO) level in given speciality by job start date (essential)

7. Completion of the application form
   - All sections of the application form completed fully (essential)

8. Clinical skills
   - Technical knowledge and clinical expertise (essential)
   - A validated logbook (essential)
   - Personal attributes (desirable)
   - Attendance of relevant courses, e.g., advanced life support (ALS), advanced trauma life support (ATLS) (desirable)

9. Academic/research skills
   - Understanding of research ± experience (essential/desirable)
   - Evidence of interest and experience of teaching (essential/desirable)
   - Evidence of research/academic achievements, e.g., prizes, publications, presentations (desirable)
   - Evidence of participation in audit (essential/desirable)
   - Evidence of participation in risk management and laboratory-based research (desirable)

10. Personal skills
    - Vigilance and situational awareness (essential)
    - Judgement/coping under pressure (essential)
    - Leadership/managing others and team involvement (essential)
    - Problem solving (essential)

- Decision making (essential)
- Empathy and sympathy (essential)
- Communication skills (essential)
- Organization and planning (essential)
- Aptitude for practical skills (desirable)

11. Probity
- Professional integrity (essential)
- Respect for others (essential)

12. Commitment to speciality
- Learning and development (essential)
- Extracurricular activities/achievements relevant to speciality (desirable).

The person specification for acute medicine (as stated on the MMC website: www.mmc.nhs.uk/default.aspx?page=326) is shown in *Table 2.1* as an example.

'Time spent abroad – does it count as training?'

Time spent abroad can be included as time in a speciality for the purposes of meeting the selection criteria. However, it is worthwhile remembering that, if this post has not been accredited as a training post, you may – following completion of specialist training – be awarded a certificate of equivalence rather than a Certificate of Completion of Training (CCT). The significance of this is that a certificate of equivalence can count against you when applying for a consultant post, as hospital trusts are well within their right to specify a CCT as essential criteria for selection.

TABLE 2.1 (*part 1*)   Person specification for acute medicine

Entry criteria	Essential	Desirable	When evaluated
Qualifications	• MBBS or equivalent medical qualification • MRCP (UK) or equivalent		Application form
Eligibility	• Eligible for full or limited registration with the GMC at time of appointment		Application form
	• Evidence of achievement of Foundation competencies by time of appointment in line with GMC standards/*Good Medical Practice* including: – good clinical care – maintaining good medical practice – good relationships and communication with patients – good working relationships with colleagues – good teaching and training – professional behaviour and probity – delivery of good acute clinical care		Application form Interview/Selection centre
	• Evidence of achievement of ST1 competencies in medicine and/or acute care specialities at time of appointment, and ST2 competencies in medicine and/or acute care specialties by August 2007		Application form Interview/Selection centre
	• Eligibility to work in the UK		Application form
Fitness to practise	• Is up-to-date and fit to practise safely		Application form References
Language skills	• All applicants to have demonstrable skills in written and spoken English that are adequate to enable effective communication about medical topics with patients and colleagues which could be demonstrated by one of the following: a) that applicants have undertaken undergraduate medical training in English or b) have the following scores in the academic International English Language Testing System (IELTS) – Overall 7, Speaking 7, Listening 6, Reading 6, and Writing 6 However, if applicants believe that they have adequate communication skills but do not fit into one of the examples they need to provide evidence		Application form Interview/Selection centre

ALS, advanced life support; APLS, advanced paediatric life support; ATLS, advanced trauma life support; EPLS, European paediatric life support.

TABLE 2.1 (*part 2*) Person specification for acute medicine

Entry criteria	Essential	Desirable	When evaluated
Health	• Meets professional health requirements (in line with GMC standards/*Good Medical Practice*)		Application form Pre-employment health screening
Career progression	• Ability to provide complete details of employment history • At least 24 months' experience (at SHO level) in medicine and/or acute care specialities (not including Foundation modules) by August 2007		Application form
Application completion	• **ALL** sections of application form **FULLY** completed according to written guidelines		Application form
Clinical skills	• **Clinical knowledge and expertise**: Appropriate knowledge base and capacity to apply sound clinical judgement to problems. Able to prioritize clinical need and aware of the basics of managing acutely ill patients. Exposure to basic practical procedures	• Attendance at relevant courses, e.g. ALS, ATLS, EPLS, APLS or equivalent	Application form Interview/Selection centre References
Academic/ research skills	• **Research skills**: Demonstrates understanding of the principles of audit and research • **Teaching**: Evidence of interest and experience in teaching • Evidence of active participation in audit	• Evidence of relevant academic and research achievements, e.g., degrees, prizes, awards, distinctions, publications, presentations, other achievements	Application form Interview/Selection centre

ALS, advanced life support; APLS, advanced paediatric life support; ATLS, advanced trauma life support; EPLS, European paediatric life support.

TABLE 2.1 (*part 3*)   Person specification for acute medicine

Entry criteria	Essential	Desirable	When evaluated
Personal skills	• **Vigilance and situational awareness**: Capacity to be alert to dangers or problems, particularly in relation to clinical governance. Capacity to monitor developing situations and anticipate issues • **Coping with pressure**: Capacity to operate under pressure. Demonstrates initiative and resilience to cope with setbacks and adapt to rapidly changing circumstances. Awareness of own limitations and when to ask for help • **Managing others and team involvement**: Capacity to work cooperatively with others and work effectively in multi-professional teams. Capacity to demonstrate leadership when appropriate, e.g., supervising junior staff • **Problem solving and decision making**: Capacity to use logical/lateral thinking to solve problems and make decisions • **Empathy and sensitivity**: Capacity to take in others' perspectives and treat others with understanding; sees patients as people • **Communication skills**: Demonstrates clarity in written/spoken communication and capacity to adapt language as appropriate to the situation. Able to build rapport, listen, persuade and negotiate • **Organization and planning**: Capacity to organize oneself, prioritize own work and organize ward rounds. Demonstrates punctuality, preparation and self-discipline. Basic IT skills	• Aptitude for practical skills	Application form Interview/Selection centre References
Probity	• **Professional integrity and respect for others**: Capacity to take responsibility for own actions and demonstrate a non-judgemental approach towards others. Displays honesty, integrity, awareness of confidentiality and ethical issues		Application form Interview/Selection centre References
Commitment to speciality	• **Learning and personal development**: Demonstrates interest and realistic insight into acute medicine. Demonstrates self-awareness and ability to accept feedback	• Extracurricular activities/ achievements relevant to acute medicine	Application form Interview/Selection centre References

ALS, advanced life support; APLS, advanced paediatric life support; ATLS, advanced trauma life support; EPLS, European paediatric life support.

Your application form

The application form for entry into specialist registrar training, regardless of speciality, pre-MMC was typically divided into three broad areas, namely:

- Clinical experience
  - Appointments to date
  - Statement of summary of clinical experience
  - Summary of logbook of procedures
  - Courses
- Interests, personal attributes and career aims
  - Teaching experience, including the teaching methods used
  - Management experience
  - Audit experience
  - Information technology (IT) experience, e.g., European computer driving license (ECDL)
  - Interests (including those outside medicine) + personal attributes
  - Career aim
- Research experience, presentations and publications
  - Academic and research experience
  - Presentations (regional, national and international)
  - Publications
  - Awards or prizes.

During Medical Training Application Service (MTAS) a number of generic questions, e.g., on teamwork or motivation, were also incorporated. The application forms for speciality training in 2008 and beyond are likely to take the form of a structured CV (similar to pre-MMC) and, in addition, may include a number of speciality-specific questions. It is important to note, however, that application forms will vary, albeit very subtly, between deaneries or speciality schools.

After application, there will be a delayed period while shortlisting occurs and then those successful candidates that are shortlisted will be asked to attend for interviews. It is *imperative* that before the interview you read your application form thoroughly and are able to expand on and discuss all aspects of your form in detail. In addition, you should also know your portfolio inside and out and, likewise, should be able to answer questions relating to it.

The process of selection

Shortlisting and longlisting

After the close of applications, there is a two-stage deanery-led process of selection (longlisting and shortlisting). The first stage (longlisting) assesses the eligibility of the applicant – i.e., whether they meet the essential criteria stated on the person specification; the second shortlists the candidate for interview. Local selection panels will perform shortlisting (stage 2) for interview locally. Those involved in shortlisting, unlike in round 1 in 2007, will be able to review the entire structured application form except for equal opportunity monitoring and personal data.

Following shortlisting, candidates will be made an offer of an interview and will be asked to confirm their intention to attend the interview within the stated time.

After the interview, which again will be conducted locally by local selection panels, candidates will be scored and ranked. Importantly, as each station/section of the interview is likely to carry the same weight, it is essential that you prepare equally for all parts. In addition to your application form, interviewers will also take into account your portfolio and the summary of your portfolio of evidence.

Tie-breaking candidates

Different deaneries will use different criteria for tie-breaking if candidates have identical scores, and usually the interviewing faculty will take a vote in order to reach a consensus.

The selection panel

The interview may be divided into stations (traditionally three) and there are typically two or three interviewers per station, one of whom will be the chairperson, with the remaining members of the interview panel asking the questions. Alternatively, there may only be one interview panel, with a chairperson and a number (as many as eight people) of other interviewers. Guidelines recommend that the interview panel should include the following members:

- A lay chair or lay representation (this can be a non-executive director, senior nurse, patient advocate, medical personnel representative or anyone not directly involved in training junior doctors or dentists)
- The regional college adviser or nominated deputy

- A university representative
- The programme director or chair of the speciality training committee (STC)
- Consultant representation from the training programme(s)
- A senior management representative.

All candidates are typically asked the same or similar questions and these are usually semi-structured. Interviewees are then scored by all members of the interview panel according to the person specification for the post, and have the opportunity to add comments to justify the score given. The highest ranked candidates will be given a job offer.

It should be possible prior to the interview to request information regarding who will be on the interview panel from the deanery, and it is always a good idea to research each panel member's speciality as well as research interests and bugbears.

Getting ahead

Mock interviews

A number of deaneries (e.g., Yorkshire Deanery) offer mock interviews, and it is worth contacting the deanery you have been shortlisted for to see if they offer such as service. Mock interviews are usually held either at the deanery or within education centres affiliated to the deanery. You should ask about the opportunity for mock interviews early as places fill rapidly.

There is no excuse for inadequate or poor preparation; and practise, practise and more practise of interview technique is undoubtedly the key to success in postgraduate interviews. You should therefore swallow your pride and ask colleagues, your educational supervisor and your consultant trainer for interview advice and, more importantly, interview practice. It is essential that you also ask for feedback regarding your performance, and this is an ideal opportunity for annoying mannerisms (e.g., finger-tapping and non-verbal body language such as playing with your hair) as well as deficiencies in your knowledge to be flagged up and put to rest. Prior to the interview you should rehearse answers to commonly asked questions and be comfortable, natural and confident with your responses.

Contact your deanery well ahead of your interview to establish the exact format of your interview. You are well within your rights to request this information. This will then guide your interview preparation.

Pre-interview visits

These are a useful opportunity to put faces to names and also find out a bit more about the job(s) and any ongoing initiatives or projects within your recruiting hospital trust. Carry out research into the recruiting hospital, trust or clinic. What is its reputation, how did it perform against its targets, and what are the issues it is facing?

You should draw up a list of questions that you want to ask before visiting, as it can potentially be embarrassing if you turn up and have nothing to ask. The general advice with regard to pre-interview visits is that, you should either visit and leave a good impression or not visit at all.

If you decide against a pre-hospital visit, you should still endeavour to find out more about the region to which you are applying – i.e., the hospitals within the rotation, their reputation, performance against targets, strengths, research interests and other issues they may be facing including merger, closure, etc.

Keep abreast of the changes

During the period of transition, it is essential that you are aware of any changes to the application system. Ensure that you check your MMC/deanery website regularly, that you have your applicant's guide fully up-to-date, including the essential and desirable person specifications, and if possible sign up to the regular email alerts/updates by the MMC communications team; this can be either via the MMC website or your relevant Royal College trainees' group, e.g., Association of Surgeons in Training (ASIT). Other useful websites include those of BMJ Careers and BMA.

Reference

General Medical Council. (2006) *Good Medical Practice*. 4E, GMC, London.

3 Your portfolio

Under Modernising Medical Careers the emphasis is on achieving competencies and a logbook of procedures/operations and references on their own are no longer sufficient. Applicants are now expected to provide proof that their educational activities are relevant and to clearly document their professional development in the form of a portfolio. This should be taken with you to the interview.

What is a portfolio?

Portfolios were initially developed in the 1940s and have been popular as a tool for assessing professional competence and proficiency in occupations such as architecture and the arts for some time. It has, however, not been until recently that they have become popular in medicine.

Due to their flexible nature and multiple components, portfolios are thought to give a more representative view of you as an individual than perhaps your CV alone. However, your portfolio is only as good as you make it and, for the purpose of the interview, it is a real gift of an opportunity for you to highlight your best attributes.

In addition to its use as a selection tool for speciality training, your portfolio should encourage you to reflect upon your achievements, identify your strengths and weaknesses, and help you to direct your future learning – i.e., it should encourage reflective learning and facilitate continued professional development (CPD). In addition, should you not make the shortlist or interview, it is a useful tool to consult in order to identify areas that could be improved upon before the next round of interviews (see *Box 3.1*).

Note: Portfolios and logbooks should be clearly labelled at the front with

---

Box 3.1 Preparing your portfolio

- Your curriculum vitae (CV)
- Exam certificates
- Certificates of course attendance
- Posters presented at learned meetings
- Presentations including at journal clubs
- Abstracts and papers (full texts)
- Audit projects (full texts)
- Your personal development plan or educational contract
- A statement of your personal values – i.e., a health and probity statement
- Record of in-training assessments (RITAs)
- Workplace based assessments (WPBAs)
  - 360-degree assessments or mini-peer assessment tools (mini-PATs)
  - Directly observed procedures (DOPs)
  - Mini-clinical evaluation exercises (mini-CEX)
  - Case-based discussions
  - Procedure-based assessments
- Appraisals
- A reflective log of activities and experience
- Logbook of clinical activity (e.g., procedures or operations) or record of achieved competencies signed by your trainer
- References (usually structured)

---

your name and GMC number, as they may be taken from you at the time of interview for review.

Online so-called e-portfolios for trainees have been developed in medicine and surgery by the respective Royal Colleges.

Your curriculum vitae

You will receive differing advice as to the format of your CV and there are no hard and fast rules. Your CV should, however, be dynamic and continuously updated as you progress through medical training and should serve not only as a job application tool but should also help guide your personal and professional development by highlighting areas in which you are deficient. In addition, for the purposes of the interview, your CV should be adapted and tailored to the post for which you are applying. Your CV is potentially the gateway to your speciality of choice and gives you an opportunity to put your best attributes forward and demonstrate that you fulfil, if not exceed, the criteria (both essential and desirable) required for the job. Your CV should serve not only as a useful reference during your interview but should also form the template for your application, and you should attempt when completing your application form to draw on as many, if not all, components of your CV.

General advice

- Use a word processor.
- Be consistent with the layout.
- Use a single font at a size which is easy to read (ideally font size 10–12).
- Avoid underlining text, and use bullets and bolding to highlight text – this is easier on the eye.
- Ensure text, bullets and especially dates are aligned.
- Check for typographical errors and spelling mistakes – use a spell- and grammar-checker.
- Use space efficiently and effectively and be succinct. Space allocated to an area should reflect its importance.
- Avoid extensive prose and the use of tables.
- Structure your CV logically, highlighting your key selling points – remember this may be the 100th CV the interview panel will have reviewed that day.
- Make sure your CV is relevant and tailored to the person specification of the post you are applying for.
- Show your CV to others to get another perspective.
- Account for any breaks in your career (you will not be penalized for this).
- Don't embellish or falsify your CV.
- Stick to the criteria, which may for example specify that your CV should be no longer than a page.

Length of your CV

Advice is conflicting as to the ideal length of your CV. In the medical specialities, shorter succinct CVs are generally preferred and in the surgical specialties, the longer the CV (not to be confused with waffley) the better. In some regards, it may be better to play it safe and have both a long version and a summary.

A 7–8 page CV is not uncommon if you are applying for an ST3 position; however, some jobs will specify the desired CV length and it is important that you stick to the specified criteria. As a rule of thumb, exclude anything from the CV that does not support the person specification for the post applied for and anything which adds little value to your application, e.g., list of meetings attended, marital status.

Your CV is an integral part of your portfolio and, importantly, your portfolio should readily display the evidence to support the achievements listed within your CV, e.g., course certificates, full text of papers/abstracts.

Suggested general format

TITLE PAGE
- Full name
- Qualifications, e.g., MBBS, MRCS, MD, BSc.

PERSONAL DETAILS
- Correspondence address
- Contact number ± fax number
- Nationality
- Gender
- Date of birth
- Current position, e.g., Clinical Research Fellow
- GMC registration number
- Medical defence organisation.

EDUCATION
- Secondary school attended
- Medical school attended
- Other universities attended.

QUALIFICATIONS
- A-level/GCSE
- University degrees with dates awarded
- Postgraduate diplomas/degrees, e.g., MRCS, MD, including dates
- Diplomas, e.g., ATLS/ALS
- Do *not* include failed exams.

CLINICAL APPOINTMENTS – list in reverse chronological order – i.e., most recent first
- Current post including dates
- Previous posts including dates.

SUMMARY OF CLINICAL EXPERIENCE – list in reverse chronological order
- Pre-medical (if any)
- Medical school, e.g., elective if relevant
- BSc or other degree
- House jobs (brief summary)
- SHO/registrar posts, e.g., table of jobs, procedures, operations.

Skills acquired should be summarized in the context of the person specification.

PRIZES/AWARDS – list in reverse chronological order
- Undergraduate and postgraduate
- Research grants/fellowships.

TEACHING EXPERIENCE
- Undergraduate, e.g., final year tutor, postgraduate, paramedical
- Practical skills teaching, e.g., anatomy demonstrating, clinical skills
- Courses organized
- Courses taught on.

RESEARCH EXPERIENCE – highlight your role and contribution
- Undergraduate, e.g., BSc
- Postgraduate
- Current projects
- Journal club attendance.

EVIDENCE OF AUDIT – highlight your role and contribution

POSITIONS OF RESPONSIBILITY
- At school
- At university
- At postgraduate level, e.g., committees.

PUBLICATIONS
- State whether abstract or full paper
- Give the full reference – use the Vancouver style
- Underline or bold your name on the reference.

PRESENTATIONS – state whether oral or poster presentation; give name of meeting, titles, authors and date.
- International
- National
- Regional
- Also invited lectures.

COURSES ATTENDED – with name, location and dates
- Undergraduate
- Postgraduate.

MEMBERSHIP OF LEARNED SOCIETIES

INTERESTS AND HOBBIES
- Don't simply list these but describe the skills that they have enabled you to develop which you can transport to clinical practice.

CAREER INTENTIONS/AIMS

REFEREES
- You should include at least two.
- One should be your current consultant and the other a previous consultant.
- You must ask your consultant before using them as a referee.
- State full name of referees, job title, address, fax and telephone number and email address.

Logbooks

A logbook is a self- or centrally-held structured record of your achievements or experiences within a particular area of medical practice (e.g., operative or interventional procedures). In the context of the interview, your logbook is used to verify and quantify your achievements to date and it should include observed as well as performed procedures.

Importantly, if you keep either personal or electronic records of patient data, you should be aware of the provisions of the Data Protection Act (1998). This requires that if data are held or recorded that can identify a patient, e.g., the patient's name, then the person responsible should be registered for this purpose under the provisions of the Data Protection Act (see www.informationcommissioner.gov.uk). Data that can only be matched to a patient with the use of additional software, e.g., patient hospital numbers, can, however, be lawfully held on a non-networked computer. Nevertheless, the general advice would be to use the information recording systems that have been developed by the relevant Royal College or training body for your speciality of interest.

Exam certificates

The original copy of all of your examination certificates to date should be incorporated within your portfolio, as evidence. Examination certificates for the following examinations are expected and essential:

- MBBS
- MRCS, MRCP, MRCGP or equivalent Royal College membership
- Intercalated BSc or honours degree
- MD, MSc or PhD.

In addition, the following could also be incorporated:

- Certificates of attendance to relevant courses, e.g., ALS, ATLS, CRISP

- Certificates of attendance at meetings, especially those that are recognized as part of training and accrue CPD points.
- Evidence of teaching on courses. If you do teach or have done so in the past, most course organizers will be able to provide you with a letter to this effect, which can be incorporated into your portfolio
- Diplomas, e.g., DRCOG, DCH.

Presentations and posters presented at learned meetings

Copies of oral (e.g., as a handout of PowerPoint slides) and poster (e.g., as a reduced size copy – ideally A4) presentations should also be included within your portfolio. These can be usefully divided into those presentations delivered at international, national, regional and hospital/trust-based (e.g., grand rounds, departmental) meetings. Remember, you should be prepared to discuss the presentations included in your portfolio in detail at interview.

Abstracts, papers and audit projects

A copy of the full text relating to all papers and conference/meeting abstracts should be included and, with respect to conference abstracts, a copy of the conference proceedings (detailing the abstract) should also be incorporated.

Audits should be written up in the style of a paper, stating the Aim, Methodology, Results, Outcome and, where appropriate, data from subsequent audits performed to complete the 'audit cycle' should also be incorporated.

Your personal development plan or educational contract

This is essentially a statement that should outline your career intentions (e.g., renal medicine, neurosurgery) and pathway, as well as what you perceive to be the endpoint of your training and how you envisage this will be achieved, e.g., 'I would like to eventually be a Consultant Anaesthetist with a specialist interest in paediatric anaesthesia. At the end of my specialist training I hope to do a fellowship abroad to gain further expertise in this area.'

A statement of personal values and aims

This should be a short (250–300 words) and concise description of your core or governing values, i.e., a summary of your beliefs. A statement of values defines how a person will act within an organization (i.e., the NHS), their interaction with colleagues and patients and, moreover, their contribution to the culture within the NHS. Your values are subjective and influenced by your life experiences and will consequently evolve over time. You should aim to include 4–6 values, taking into consideration patients, the medical community/institution and colleagues. In terms of the use of statements of value, the interviewer will be looking for values that are congruous or will enhance the corporate culture within their institution. Values that could be used include ambition, individuality, integrity, dedication, fun, loyalty, honesty, innovativeness, teamwork, excellence, efficiency, dignity, collaboration, empathy, accomplishment, friendliness, discipline/order, dependability, flexibility; however, the list is extensive.

In addition to a statement of values, you should also include a statement of your career aims within your portfolio. This is a summary of your career intentions, both in the immediate future (i.e., next 6 months) – for example, completion of postgraduate exams, attainment of competencies, e.g., in gastroscopy – as well as in the longer term (i.e., years).

Records of in-training assessment

The record of in-training assessment (RITA) was developed in 1997, following the Calman review. It is an annual summative review of the documented progress (typically using logbooks and local assessment as evidence) and performance of a trainee, which is organized by the trainee-specific Speciality Training Committee (STC). It traditionally only applies to trainees holding a national or visiting training number (NTN/VTN), or fixed term training number (FTN), or locum appointment for training (LAT); however, it is starting to be rolled out for ST1/ST2 trainees.

The outcome of the RITA review is recorded as either RITA C – trainee is making satisfactory progress, RITA D – a minor correctable problem has been identified and the trainee requires targeted training, or RITA E – a more major problem is identified and the trainee requires targeted additional training, as determined by the postgraduate dean.

The purpose of the RITA is to ensure that trainees receive educational guidance and to identify and address their educational needs throughout their training. The documented outcome if you have previously undertaken a RITA should be included within your portfolio.

Workplace based assessments

Workplace based assessments (WPBAs) form an integral part of the assessment of competency of trainees. They not only ensure that trainees progress satisfactorily, but also provide documented evidence of learning and development. The principles for assessment and guidance on workplace based assessment are established by the Postgraduate Medical Education and Training Board (PMETB).

Workplace based assessments is a term that embraces a spectrum of assessment tools including: 360-degree assessments or mini-peer assessment tool (mini-PAT); mini-clinical evaluation exercise (mini-CEX); directly observed procedures (DOPs); case-based discussions (CBDs) and procedure-based assessments (PBAs). The underlying principle is that trainees are assessed on work that they actually perform and thus the assessment is integrated into the trainee's day-to-day work. For WPBA to be effective, the method of assessment must be robust (quality assured), reliable, valid and fit for purpose, and trainees should:

- Understand the purpose of the assessment
- Be given formative feedback following assessment, which will inform and guide their personal development
- Be assessed by a number of different assessors or trainers
- Be assessed over a broad range of activities, using a number of different 'assessment tools', e.g., those in Foundation training are expected to undertake a minimum of 20 assessments.

Workplace based assessment is 'trainee led' and it is up to the trainee to identify suitable opportunities and decide when, where and who will assess them, with the guidance of their educational supervisor. Anyone competent in performing the assessed competency may act as an assessor. Each encounter should typically take 15 minutes and a further 5 minutes is then devoted to meaningful formative feedback. Each assessment is scored using a structured tick-list form, and a copy is held by the trainee as part of the body of evidence of satisfactory progression contained within the trainee's (electronic) learning portfolio, which will be subject to annual review.

Types of work-based assessment

Mini-peer assessment tool or 360-degree assessments

The 360-degree assessment, otherwise known as the mini-PAT or multi-source feedback (MSF), is a concept that originated from the commercial sector and is a process whereby evidence regarding your performance at work is gathered from a number of different co-workers (typically between 8 and 12). The list should be agreed with your educational supervisor and may include medical colleagues (of different grades), your educational supervisor, secretarial or clerical staff, biomedical scientists, nurses, pharmacists, etc., and in some specialities it may be appropriate to involve patients – the theory being that by taking a 'multi-source' approach, a more holistic and objective view of you as a doctor within a team-working environment can be achieved. 360-Degree assessments are thought to more fair compared to the traditional single-source reference, which has the potential of being open to bias.

Methods that can be used in formal 360-degree appraisal may include unstructured interviews, statements with a simple rating scale and, more commonly, structured questionnaires using indicators of good performance, as determined by *Good Medical Practice* (GMC 2006) and Royal College speciality curricula. The information is then gathered, analyzed and the results constructively fed back anonymously to the appraisee/trainee by the trainee's educational supervisor and used to guide their personal development. It is likely that the mini-PAT assessment will be undertaken every 3 years in speciality training, e.g., at ST1, ST4 and ST7; where a problem is identified, it may be used more frequently.

For the purposes of your portfolio at interview, in addition to your mini-PAT, you could include additional 'multi-source' evidence in the form of 'thank you' letters from patients or letters recognizing your contribution to aspects of your working life, e.g., mess president, rota development, etc.

Mini-clinical evaluation exercise (mini-CEX)

The mini-clinical evaluation exercise is a method of assessing professional skills such as history taking, physical examination, clinical judgement, communicating results or discussing management with patients, professionalism, presentation skills, involvement in multidisciplinary team (MDT) meetings and others skills essential for good clinical care, as determined by the speciality specific curriculum, within the work setting.

Assessors do not need to have prior knowledge of the trainee; however, they should be competent in the area being assessed. Their evaluation is recorded on a structured checklist and constructive verbal feedback is given to the trainee immediately following assessment/the encounter. The whole process should take between 15 and 20 minutes.

Directly observed procedures (DOPs)

Direct observation of procedures is a concept initially developed by the UK Royal College of Physicians, which aims to assess competency – i.e., ability to perform a practical skill or part or all of a practical procedure within the work setting (e.g., on the ward, in outpatients, in theatre). The practical competencies assessed will be determined by the trainee's level and also their speciality. For example, at Foundation, index competencies listed on the curriculum include venesection, cannulation, blood culture, urethral catheterization and intubation.

The process of assessment is trainee-led and it is therefore up to the trainee to identify opportunities for assessment, a process which should typically take between 15 and 20 minutes. The assessors can be any healthcare professional (e.g., SpR, nurse, consultant, pharmacist) competent in performing the assessed skill and they do not necessarily have to have prior knowledge of the trainee.

Following performance of the task the assessor should give the trainee immediate feedback and their evaluation is documented on a structured checklist form, which is returned to the trainee and a copy is retained for the trainee's portfolio.

Case-based discussions (CBDs)

Case-based discussion (CBD) is a structured in-depth interview, designed to assess a trainee's clinical judgement, decision-making skills, ability to prioritize and application of medical knowledge, through discussion of a challenging clinical case managed by the trainee. This should include a detailed discussion of the actions taken, as well as any ethical and legal considerations, e.g., record keeping.

The CBD tool can be applied to both hospital and GP settings and the assessor should be a senior colleague, e.g., GP trainer, SpR or consultant. Assessments should take between 15 and 20 minutes and following completion of the assessment form (which may only be performed on-line), immediate and structured feedback should be given, which would normally take about 5 minutes. Case-based discussion essentially formalizes a well-established practice of presenting and discussing clinical cases by trainees and couples it with formal feedback. At Foundation level the criteria for assessment include: medical record keeping; clinical assessment; investigations and referrals; treatment; follow-up and future planning; professionalism and overall clinical judgement.

Procedure-based assessment (PBA)

Procedure-based assessment (PBA) is a tool that is not dissimilar from directly observed procedures (DOPs); however, it is specific to the surgical specialities. The aim of PBA is to assess the 'technical ability and professional skills' of the trainee in a range of index procedures or parts of procedures, as appropriate to the level of the trainee. The assessor following the procedure, using an assessment form that outlines both the desirable and undesirable behaviours, will be required to provide the trainee with constructive feedback which will guide future practice. The ultimate standard is that achieved for the Certificate of Completion of Training (CCT).

Reflective logs of activities and experience

Reflective practice is a concept which was initially coined in the 1980s by Donald Schön and is defined as a continuous process which involves 'thoughtfully considering one's own experiences in applying knowledge to practice while being coached by professionals in the discipline' (Schön 1983).

In essence, reflective practice can be seen as a form of experimental learning. It requires the analysis of past experiences or performances, critique of these events with the identification of aspects that were done well, as well as those that could be improved upon, with the aim of adapting your approach for future situations. The process of 'reflection' can occur 'in action' (i.e., immediately) whilst performing the task, or 'on action' (i.e., at a later stage).

Within your portfolio you should be able to demonstrate reflective learning and/or practice and this can easily be achieved in the form of a structured short statement. This should include the following:

- The setting, e.g., where, people involved, etc.
- What your role was
- The outcome
- What aspects were done well
- What aspects could be improved upon
- How you would tackle the same/similar situations in the future.

References

General Medical Council. (2006) *Good Medical Practice*. 4E, GMC, London.
Schön D.A. (1983) *The Reflective Practitioner: How Professionals Think in Action*. Temple Smith, London.

4 The interview

What to take

First impressions in any interview are very important. It is essential to be well presented and any evidence that you may need to produce during the interview should be easily accessible.

You should receive information from your deanery as to what you should take to interview. In accordance with the NHS Pre- and Post-Appointments Checks Direction 2002 and Section 8 of the Asylum and Immigration Act 1996, the deanery is required to verify your identity, registration, qualifications and status with respect to working. The following are usually required and it is worth packing these well in advance of the day:

- Proof of identity, e.g., passport or official photo ID (original + two photocopies of those pages showing your name and signature).
- Two recent, passport-type photographs with your name written clearly on the back of each.
- Your original GMC certificate for the current year + two copies.
- Your original degree certificate and relevant postgraduate qualifications including evidence of all qualifications listed on your application form, including official translations if the original is not in English (original + two copies).
- Verified evidence of competences, e.g., logbook, cited on your application form + two copies.
- Evidence of educationally approved posts as cited on your application form + two copies. This evidence can be in the form of letters of appointment to a training post or a training rotation from the relevant hospital, trust or postgraduate dean. Importantly, prior to applying for a post you should check that the posts you have previously undertaken have educational approval.

- Evidence of eligibility to take up employment in the UK, including evidence of immigration status if a non-UK/EEA applicant, or appropriate passport, birth certificate or naturalization papers for UK/EEA applicants + two copies.
- Signed/verified references + two copies (required in 2007).
- Occupational Smart Card.

If for any reason you cannot provide the above/required documents, (or a certified copy), you should contact the deanery well ahead of your interview, as failure to produce any of the requested documents on the day, may result in you not being interviewed.

Other documents, which should be taken to interview, include:

- Your curriculum vitae (CV)
- Your logbook.

These, along with any other evidence you wish to present, should be contained within your portfolio, which should be neat and in order.

In addition to the above, you may also be required to bring equipment such as a stethoscope, cranial nerve examination equipment, etc.

Take additional copies of your CV

The panel members will already have a copy of your completed application form and will request a copy of your curriculum vitae. You should have this readily available in your portfolio and it would appear more organized if you hand a copy of your curriculum vitae to the panel members before sitting down.

Claiming travel expenses

It should be possible to claim travelling expenses for attending the interview. Expense forms should be available at interview and some deaneries ask for confirmation that you will be claiming for travel expenses in advance. Others may require a request in writing, especially if overnight accommodation is required. Costs are paid in accordance with the Whitley Council Terms and Conditions and receipts for costs incurred will need to be produced.

What to expect and interview styles

The most common form of postgraduate medical interview nowadays is a structured interview, usually with three stations and two panel members in each station; however, there are variations to this. For instance, there may be two stations with two or three panel members at each station or there may be three stations with three panel members at each and there may even be additional stations, e.g., four or five.

Each station will last a minimum of 10 minutes and different interview styles may be used in the different stations. In some stations one panel member may ask all of the questions but both will mark separately and in other stations one panel member may ask questions for the first 5 minutes and then they will change over so that the other panel member asks the questions for the second 5 minutes. You should expect to cover three or four questions within each station. Importantly, these questions are usually not varied between candidates, so it really is in your best interest not to divulge questions to candidates awaiting interview on the same day.

In a structured interview the stations are based upon a person's specification. There will undoubtedly be a station related to clinical experience and a second station related to research, audit, publications and presentations. The third station may be variable.

At some interviews, the interviewer may systematically take you through your portfolio, discussing the evidence contained within it. For instance, you may have a case-based discussion or a procedure-based assessment, which the interviewer will select and discuss with you in depth. Courses or conferences that you have attended may also be selected out and discussed in this station. Many feel that a portfolio station is not discriminatory and some trainees have felt that the time has not allowed them to fully justify everything that they have done, but it is up to you to try to bring out the best in your portfolio.

In other interviews the final station may take the form of a discussion on issues, such as management and clinical governance. Whatever the format, the stations of the interview in total will cover the whole of the person specification for that post.

Marking the candidate

In each station each panel member will mark the sections discussed in that station separate to his/her co-panel member. There will therefore be two sets of marks at least for each station.

If you feel you have done particularly badly in one station you should try to put it behind you in the time between stations. Remember that the next panel does not know how you have just performed and it is quite possible that you may not have performed as badly as you think you did. You should go into the remaining stations, remembering that you still have a chance of redeeming yourself.

Commonly encountered scenarios and questions will be discussed in further detail in subsequent chapters.

Other types of interview

Increasingly, deaneries are becoming more adventurous and newer forms of evaluation are being introduced in an attempt to make the interview process fairer and to more globally assess a candidate. For 2008, communication skills and practical skills (see below) will not normally be present but some specialities may have these. From 2009 onwards, these types of station will become more commonplace.

Alternative forms of evaluation/assessment include:

- *Presentations*: These are widely used at entry at specialist registrar and consultant level. Candidates will be advised of the topic of their presentation at the time of notification of the interview. Topics are varied and can be medical/clinical, where the emphasis is often placed on medical ethics or the multi-disciplinary approach to patient care, or non-medical, where the emphasis is commonly on team building, management, problem solving and communication skills. All shortlisted candidates will be given the same topic, so the panel may very well have heard the same/similar presentation several times over by the time yours is heard, so try to make your presentation different, dynamic and to the point, but most of all keep to time.
- *Objective structured clinical examinations* (*OSCEs*): see section on *Assessment of practical skills at interview* in chapter 7.
- *Critical analysis*: Candidates may be asked to critically appraise (read, interpret and summarize) a medical or even a non-medical paper prior to the interview and to either present or discuss the paper at interview.
- *Assessment of communication skills*: This can take the form part of an OSCE with the use of actors/patients and scenarios that are commonly encountered in clinical practice, e.g., consent for a procedure, an outpatient clinic, breaking bad news, dealing with difficult patients/colleagues, etc.
- *Psychometric testing*: This was trialled as a mode of assessment by the East of England Deanery in 2007 and its cost–benefit is still being evaluated. The Meyers–Briggs test is the mostly widely recognized and applied psychometric test.

General interview tips for on the day

- An interview coordinator will call you well before your interview time to collect the required documentation.
- Arrive early for the interview so that you have plenty of time to prepare yourself and hand in the necessary documentation. It does not reflect well if you arrive short of breath and sweating, having just run up the road. If you are running late, you should try to telephone through as it may be possible to reorganize the timings of the interview. If you just turn up late, then you may end up not being interviewed.
- Be positive and confident (not overconfident) – you have been called to interview so you have a clear and real chance at securing the job.
- At the beginning of the interview the panel members will introduce themselves to you and often will offer a handshake.
- Listen carefully to the question asked and ensure that you understand the question. If you do not understand a question, ask the interviewer to repeat it or repeat the question back to the interviewer to check that you have interpreted the question correctly. Be careful, however; this should be done only once or twice during the interview and it can annoy some interviewers.
- Don't rush into answering a question. When you hear a question, if it is something that you can answer easily and you are prepared, take a second or two before you start. It is often the first sentence that leads the discussion relating to that part of the interview and it is surprising how many people, even though they know that subject matter very well, start badly and are never able to recover.
- Answer the question! Don't go off on a tangent or answer the question that you would have liked them to ask you.
- Be honest in your response to questions. The panel are looking to employ a future colleague, and enthusiasm, commitment and honesty can by far replace any deficiencies that you feel you have.
- Direct your response to the person asking the question, but make sure you don't ignore the rest of the panel.
- Avoid sounding as though you have rote-learnt answers to questions. Even if you have a well-rehearsed response to a question, pause and deliver your reply in keeping with your personality – i.e., as naturally as possible.
- When answering questions, use 'I' rather than 'we'. The former has greater impact and is generally associated with greater accountability.
- You can to some extent control the direction of the interview. If there are particular areas that you would like to be questioned on, finish your response to your last question by alluding to this area. The interviewer may or may not take the bait. You should not do this with every question.

- Throughout the interview maintain good eye contact with all members of the panel.
- Avoid fidgeting – placing your hands firmly on your knees throughout the interview often helps.
- During the interview you may hear bells or knocks on the door indicating the times. Do not be put off by these. Keep talking until someone tells you that the interview has finished.
- At the end of the interview, you may be asked whether you have any questions (you will not be penalized for not having any questions). Your options in response to this question include:
  - Politely say 'no' (the safest option).
  - Politely say 'no', and allude to the fact that all your questions were answered during your pre-interview visit.
  - Ask a question. Beware, however, that the question has not been answered elsewhere, (e.g., in the person specification) or that it demonstrates ignorance.
- In addition at the end of the interview, you may be asked whether you have anything further that you would like to add in support of your application and this is a valuable opportunity to flag up any attributes, skills or achievements that have not been covered in the course of the interview which are relevant. Remember, this may be your one and only bite of the cherry. Now is not the time to be modest about your achievements. If you don't sell your qualities, nobody else will.
- At the end of the interview, you should be courteous and say thank you and should remember to collect your portfolio before leaving. You will initially be asked by the interview coordinator to wait outside and will then be directed to your next station.
- Once you have finished all of the stations you will be allowed to leave the interview area.
- Finally, try to enjoy the interview and remember to smile.

Common interview myths

You do not need to prepare for an interview

Interviews should be considered very much like an examination. It is an in-depth discussion about your career to date and often about how you see things in the future. It requires a lot of preparation. You should know your CV inside and out and, in addition, you should be able to discuss the posts that you have already undertaken, why you undertook them and what experience you gained from them. You will also be expected to discuss in detail any operations or practical procedures that you may have performed or observed and, of course, any academic research that you have been involved with or publications that you produced are quite likely to be scrutinized.

The panel members are unprepared

This is far from the truth. All the members of the interview panel will have met with the lay-chairman 30–45 minutes before the interviews start. It will be decided who is in which station and the panel members will decide what questions they are going to ask and they will discuss this with their co-panel member to ensure that the question is easy to understand and is a fair discriminator. Although there will be variation in the way the questions are put forward, there will be a common theme to each. Many of the questions will relate to clinical scenarios, and this in particular holds true for the station relating to clinical governance and management.

References play an important part in the interview process

This is not correct. The references are often not even seen by the panel members but are viewed only by the lay-chairman. A major role of the lay-chairman is to review the written references and to ensure that there is nothing in a reference which would deem that person unappointable. If the lay-chairman finds something in a reference that the panel members may need to probe in more detail, this will be made known to the panel members so that they can discuss the particular area raised within the reference during the interview. For the vast majority of people, their references are ticked off as satisfactory by the lay-chairman.

In addition to checking the references the lay-chairman is also responsible for checking that the candidate has met all the eligibility criteria, e.g., number of months' experience, and even at the stage of the interview issues about eligibility can be raised.

Importantly, if your references are outstanding at the time of your interview you may be penalized – i.e., scored down. It is your responsibility to make sure that this is not the case and you should contact your referees prior to the interview to check that they have completed and submitted references.

References can be unstructured (free text) or be structured. In the latter your referee may be asked a number of questions including those regarding your clinical ability, future potential, team-working skills and interaction with patients and colleagues – those attributes as outlined by the GMC's document *Good Medical Practice* (GMC 2006).

The person for the job has already been decided or this region only ever takes its own trainees

With greater transparency in the selection process, the days of consultants exclusively 'looking after their own' has gone. By virtue of the fact that you have been shortlisted for interview means that you are clearly in the running for the job and you should go into the interview confident and positive, as your performance on the day will be the determining factor.

What you wear and your body language are not important

All panel members at an interview will have been through a course on how to interview. Part of that course includes discussion on how to eliminate biases and although theoretically your appearance and body language should not affect the outcome of the interview, the interviewer will formulate an opinion about the interviewee during the first minute of the interview and human nature dictates that your presentation will inevitably influence this opinion. Dressing smartly, a pleasant greeting at the beginning and a comfortable posture while sitting during the interview all help to make the process much more relaxing and gives a good impression. In addition, speak slowly and clearly. Monosyllabic answers are no good in an interview that is trying to probe in depth and you should expect many parts of the interview to be a two-way discussion.

Dress code for interviews is smart and conservative. Men should wear suits with ties and women similarly should wear suits/jackets.

An interview is only about the CV, it has got nothing to do with knowledge

This is a common myth and many people go into the interview unprepared and not expecting clinical or basic science type questions. Not surprisingly, if you are not prepared for these types of question, you will be totally thrown by them when they are asked and will therefore perform poorly overall.

It should be remembered, however, that the vast majority of the questions will be related to the person specification and the evidence that you contain in your portfolio. You have no excuse for not preparing for these types of question in advance of the interview.

The panel are trying to trick and fail you

This is not the way an interview panel works. The panel members are trying to find out as much about you as they can during the time allotted. They are not trying to trick you and there will be no trick questions. Of course they may be dissatisfied with some of your answers. If you do not agree with the interviewer, you are at liberty during the interview to express your opinion. However, it is always much better if you can back up this opinion with some evidence, and you should not get into a full blown argument because usually the interviewer will almost always be right.

The interviewers discuss your performance after you have left

With a structured interview this does not occur. There is no time for any discussion because by the time each interviewer has scored each section that they have interviewed on, the next candidate is ready to come in. This should remove any bias and, of course, gives the candidate at least a double mark (depending on the number or interviewers, i.e., may be more) for each section that they have been through.

The panel members can change their marks after the interview

After the interviews have been completed, all the marks for each of the candidates are collated and added up and, as a result of this, the candidates are ranked. It is not possible for the marks to be changed as they are collected from the panel members by the administrative coordinator at regular intervals during the interviews and are collated into the accumulated scores. In the briefing discussion before the interviews begin, the panel members may decide that certain questions are so important that should a candidate not answer them correctly they will be 'red-carded'. This often relates to clinical scenarios where the panel may feel that the candidate's clinical experience, if they could not answer the question appropriately, would deem them unsuitable for the post for which they were being interviewed. Before the interviews the panel members and the lay-chairman discuss the issue of 'red-carding' and establish clear guidelines as to the grounds on which a 'red card' can be issued. Thus, after the interview when the marks are looked at, although a candidate may have been ranked high enough to be offered a job, if they have been 'red-carded' in any section of the interview, they will be automatically eliminated from the selection.

Reference

General Medical Council. (2006) *Good Medical Practice*. 4E, GMC, London.

5 Hot interview topics

There is a large amount of preparation required to undertake an interview successfully. Part of your preparation should be spent going over questions that are commonly asked and preparing answers to each question according to your own experience.

This book has been designed to help you think about the answers; it is not designed or intended to give you model answers, nor would the authors wish this. It attempts, however, to give you a basic understanding of common topics and a framework onto which to hang your answers.

There may be some differences between specialities as to the type of questions asked and the type of answers expected, particularly when one considers the craft specialities. Most interviews are divided into the following broad categories:

1. Academic research, teaching and publications
2. Clinical governance, audit and management (this may be replaced by a portfolio-based interview)
3. Curriculum vitae, clinical experience, motivation and personality
4. Portfolio-based interviews (if this station is included).

In addition, there are also likely to be a large number of generic questions.

Helpful pointers

- The interview is your chance to sell your qualities and to convince the interview panel that you are the best person for the job.
- Responses should be structured and thoughtful. Where appropriate, use your own experiences as evidence that you have the essential and desirable person specifications for the job.

- If you are asked to give an opinion, it is useful to initially give both sides of the argument. However, don't sit on the fence; give an opinion one way or the other on the topic. You will undoubtedly be challenged and you should be able to defend your stance, whilst demonstrating an ability to listen to other perspectives.
- Where possible/appropriate you should try to demonstrate reflective practice, e.g., when asked to describe a situation, structure your response by giving some information regarding the setting, describe your involvement and the skills you called upon, and reflect on the outcome in terms of what you have learnt from the experience and how you may tackle the same or similar situation in the future.
- If a question/station does go badly, try and put it behind you and importantly remain calm. The odds are that you haven't done as badly as you feel you have. More importantly, you can make up lost ground in the remainder of the interview.

Academic research, publications and teaching

Academic achievements of any form – i.e., higher degrees, prizes at medical school, peer-reviewed publications and research experience – score highly. Questions here will relate to research experience, publications, presentations and teaching in general. This section may or may not also contain audit, which we will be dealing with in the section 'Clinical governance, audit and management'.

Academic research

Discussion in this part of the interview will relate to any academic research that you have previously conducted or are currently performing. Many trainees will have completed an intercalated BSc or a BSc before entering medical school. Others may have done an MSc, performed research as part of their elective or may be part way through an MD, MS or PhD at the time of their interview. In preparation, you should read up thoroughly on everything that you have done, even if it was some years ago, as this part of the interview should be unfaltering.

A common opening question is, 'Tell us about your research experience.' Although a seemingly straightforward question, it is easy to answer poorly. You should structure your answer, giving a chronological and clear description of your experience to date.

If you mention laboratory-based research you will be asked about laboratory methods and, in preparation, you should refamiliarize yourself with these. Be clear exactly what part you played in any research and if you did not personally undertake any aspects of it (e.g., laboratory experiments), then you should tell the interviewer which aspects you did and did not perform.

In addition, if research has been done but has not been presented or published, then there will need to be some acknowledgement as to why this has not occurred.

In preparing for this section you should also plan answers to questions that are likely to lead on from here. For example, 'How has this research impacted on clinical practice?' or 'What have you gained from your research?' or 'How has research helped your career development?'

If you have no experience of research, don't panic. You have been shortlisted which would imply that for this particular post at least research experience is not an important prerequisite. You may, however, be asked, 'What different types of research do you know about?' or 'Why is research important?'

Publications

Presentations and publications will, in the main, be derived from research that you have conducted, but for some they will be derived from individual case reports, audit or retrospective analysis of data. When completing the application form you should read the section on publications very carefully. Although it may fill the space on the form, some interviewers get very irritated when they see a list of publications including abstracts and letters or papers that are either in press or submitted. The experienced interviewer will not be fooled or impressed as they know that the vast majority of these will never ever be published. Interviewers want to know about the publications that have actually been accepted or those that have actually been published. Letters to a journal and abstracts should not be put under this section, but should come under a separate section on publications of letters and abstracts.

You are likely to be asked, 'Out of all of your publications, which one has been the most important?' or 'which one has made the greatest contribution?' You should ideally choose to discuss the paper to which you have contributed the most. In answering this question, you should also acknowledge to the panel the level of your contribution, although this will often be reflected in the order of authorship – i.e., whether you are first author, second author, third author, etc. Even if you have not performed the work yourself, you should have a clear understanding of all aspects of the research, including the more complex parts of the project, e.g., cell culture, RNA extraction, etc., and any question related to your area of publication will be fair game.

Finally, if your research has been presented and you did not make the presentation but were the principal author of the research, then you should explain why someone else made the presentation.

Common research-related questions

'What is research?'

The aim of research is to create new knowledge. In medical *research* (aka biomedical research or experimental medicine) the primary intention is to advance knowledge to improve patient care and its associated activities. An individual patient may or may not benefit directly.

Medical research can be categorized as *preclinical* (i.e., geared to the development of new treatments) or *clinical* (i.e., aimed at evaluating the efficacy and safety of new treatments).

'How has your research affected your clinical practice?'

Research, publications and presentations assist us in the management of patients and you need to be able to critically appraise the work you have done and whether it is something that may or has realistically altered clinical practice.

Although you are not expected to have made a groundbreaking discovery with your research, you should be able to talk fluently about your research project as well as answer related questions.

The discussion may progress onto the skills you have acquired during research and those you will carry into clinical practice, namely:

- An understanding and hands-on experience of developing a research project – i.e., methodology, ethics, understanding of statistics and data analysis, etc.
- Exposure to an academic department ± opportunities to collaborate
- Improved understanding of a particular field/subspeciality of medicine
- Furthering medical knowledge
- An appreciation of evidence-based medicine (EBM); bridging the gap between academia and clinical practice
- An ability to critically appraise papers
- The ability to work independently, think laterally, troubleshoot and self-direct learning, as well as work as part of a team
- Skills in presenting, writing and IT (information technology)
- Greater publication opportunities
- Facilitation of an academic career ± improved future job prospects.

Disadvantages of a period in research include:

- Break from clinical practice, perceived loss of clinical skills
- Lack of funding, poor recruitment, prolonging period in research
- Poor supervision, lack of support (e.g., administrative, IT)
- Isolation, bullying and harassment.

'When should doctors undertake research?'

There are no rights or wrongs to this question. This is a personal decision and doctors should ideally be given the flexibility to decide when or if at all. Research is typically undertaken at medical school in the form of a BSc or MB PhD, and in recent years has been a prerequisite to obtaining a national training number (NTN). It is debatable, however, as to whether research would be better undertaken towards the end of speciality training, if at all.

'How do you organize a research project?'

Define the aim of the project; establish a hypothesis, and methodology ± power calculations ± define randomization and blinding protocols; obtain ethical approval; collect data; perform statistical analyses, interpret results and draw appropriate conclusions. (See also the Research section in Further reading.)

'How would you introduce a new procedure or technique into clinical practice?'

The National Institute for Health and Clinical Excellence (NICE) is responsible for determining whether an interventional procedure is 'safe enough and works well enough to be used routinely or whether special arrangements are needed for patients' consent'.

An interventional procedure is defined by NICE as any procedure 'used for diagnosis and treatment which involves either making a cut or a hole to gain access to the inside of a patient's body' or one 'gaining access to a body cavity without cutting into the body, e.g., endoscopy'.

NICE has taken this role over from the Safety and Efficacy Register for New Interventional Procedures (SERNIP) – a non-governmental medical advisory body with a remit to promote sound scientific development of new procedures, which is now disbanded.

Further research-related questions

- How does research fit into the NHS?
- Why is research important?
- Should all doctors undertake a period of research?
- Can you tell me about one of your publications?
- How has your research impacted on clinical practice?

Other key areas within this section

Evidence-based medicine

Questions on evidence-based medicine (EBM) are common and your answer should be tailored to the speciality to which you are applying.

You may be asked, 'What is evidence-based medicine?' or 'Do you practice evidence-based medicine?' You should try not to just give the standard definition as, in the heat of the interview, you may very well forget the exact wording. Also, to the trained interviewer, it merely demonstrates your ability to regurgitate ready-made answers and not necessarily your understanding of the subject. Instead, you should adapt the definition to include an example specific to your speciality, e.g., the UK Small Aneurysm Trial which guides the operative management of asymptomatic abdominal aortic aneurysms.

Definition

> 'Evidence based medicine is the conscientious, explicit, and judicious use of current best evidence in making decisions about the care of individual patients. The practice of evidence based medicine means integrating individual clinical expertise with the best available external clinical evidence from systematic research.' (Sackett et al. 1996)

A common further question may be, 'What do you understand by levels of evidence?' Evidence can be classified according to its strength and freedom from bias into five hierarchical levels, level 1 being the strongest evidence and level 5 the weakest evidence (*Table 5.1*). You do not need to memorize all of the different components of each level but you should have an overview of the requirements for each.

TABLE 5.1   Evidence-based medicine: levels of evidence

Level of evidence	Type of evidence
1a	Systematic review of multiple, well-designed randomized control trials (RCTs)
1b	Individual RCT
1c	All-or-none case series
2a	Systematic review of cohort studies
2b	Individual cohort study or low-quality RCT
2c	Outcomes study, audit or ecological study
3a	Systematic review of case control studies
3b	Individual case control study
4	Case series and poor quality cohort and case control studies
5	Opinions of respected authorities based on clinical evidence, descriptive studies or reports of expert consensus committees

Common evidence-based medicine-related questions

'What are the steps involved in developing evidence-based medicine?'

There are essentially four steps to evidence-based medicine:

1. Identifying an answerable clinical question
2. Accessing information which will help to answer the question
3. Appraising the validity and relevance of the information available
4. Harnessing the information and applying it to everyday clinical practice.

'What are the advantages of evidence-based medicine?'

1. Is an objective method of determining and maintaining high quality and safety standards in medical practice
2. Facilitates transfer of clinical research into practice
3. Potentially reduces healthcare costs ± improves utilization of resources
4. Enables clinicians to improve their knowledge
5. Provides a framework for problem-solving and teaching
6. Improves computer literacy, data appraisal and interpretation, and understanding of research

7. Allows better communication with patients regarding the rationale behind treatments.

'What are the disadvantages of evidence-based medicine?'

1. Time consuming
2. Framework or resources for practising evidence-based medicine are not always available, e.g., funding
3. Not all electronic databases are comprehensive, well indexed or continuously updated
4. Older doctors may not be as computer literate and may struggle.

'What is evidence-based clinical practice?'

> 'Evidence based clinical practice is an approach to decision making in which the clinician uses the best evidence available, in consultation with the patient, to decide upon the option which suits that patient best.' (Muir Gray 1997)

'Give an example where you have practised evidence-based medicine.'

Examples could include: surgical intervention for abdominal aortic aneurysm repair – i.e., when size >5.5 cm (UK Small Aneurysm Trial); maintainance of tight glycaemic control post-myocardial infarction (DIGAMI trial); the use of clopidogrel in the secondary prevention of ischaemic events (CAPRIE trial); use of simvastatin in patients with symptomatic coronary disease (Scandinavian Simvastatin Survival Study – 4S).

'Can you tell me about a paper you have read recently that has made an impact on your clinical practice?'

Evidence-based medicine is integral to the way most clinicians will approach their clinical practice and, of course, within this part of the interview, you may be asked to describe papers and publications that have clearly altered the clinical management of patient subgroups. Within your speciality you should be aware of at least a handful of papers that are highly important and influence patient management, e.g., in vascular surgery, the UK Small Aneurysm Trial (UK SAT), General Anaesthesia versus Local Anaesthesia for Carotid Endarterectomy (GALA) Trial and EndoVascular Aneurysm Repair (EVAR) Trials I and II.

You do not need to know these publications in great detail or necessarily in which journal they were published or even when they were published. If you do, it's a bonus, but the interview panel would be quite happy to discuss these papers merely by their title.

'How do you make sure you keep up-to-date?'

In summary, this may be achieved through:

- Attending courses and conferences
- Regularly completing on-line study modules
- Reading relevant journals
- Organizing or attending and actively participating in journal club meetings. (*Note:* You may be asked to comment on a paper recently discussed.)
- Teaching peers, junior colleagues and other healthcare professionals
- Examinations, e.g., USMLE, diplomas
- Other activities that lead to the accrual of continued professional development (CPD) points.

For a useful link, see the Essential Evidence Plus website: www.infopoems.com/concept/ebm_loe.cfm.

'What is COREC (Central Office for Research Ethics Committees)?'

Ethics and ethics committees may form part of the discussion during the academic station or under the clinical governance and management station; you should have a clear understanding of the ethical considerations as well as mechanisms of quality assurance in place to safeguard research.

COREC is the Central Office for Research Ethics Committees. As well as advising and giving overall ethical approval for the research to be conducted, COREC also advises and will need to approve any explanatory paperwork that the patient will receive in order to decide whether or not they will participate in the study. This includes any correspondence that will be sent to the GP and draft copies of these letters for recruitment and consent will need to be presented to the ethics panel before approval.

In addition to COREC, each individual NHS trust will have an ethics committee that will consider in detail any proposals of research involving patients and healthy volunteers.

If you have been involved with research, it would be advisable before your interview to obtain a copy of the submission form from your ethics committee and read it carefully, in particular with respect to the requirements. Failing this, the NHS Research Ethics Committee application form can be downloaded from the internet (see www.corecform.org.uk).

'What is UK Clinical Research Collaboration (UKCRC)?'

The UK Clinical Research Collaboration (UKCRC), UK Clinical Research Network (UKCRN) and Office for Strategic Coordination of Health Research (OSCHR) are organizations which play a key role in research strategy in the UK. Although you are not expected to know about them in great detail, you should at least be aware of their existence.

The UK Clinical Research Collaboration (UKCRC; www.ukcrc.org) is an alliance of organizations with the shared aim 'to re-engineer the environment in which clinical research is conducted in the UK, to benefit the public and patients by improving national health and increasing national wealth'. It achieves this goal through developing:

- The research infrastructure and research workforce
- Incentives to conduct research in the NHS
- Clearer channels through the governance and regulatory red-tape
- A unified approach to the funding of research by government bodies.

The UK Clinical Research Network (UKCRN) is part of the UKCRC and was designed in order 'to support the conduct of high quality clinical trials and other well designed studies'.

The Office for Strategic Coordination of Health Research (OSCHR) was established following Sir David Cooksey's review into the public funding of UK health research in 2006 and its role is to 'take the lead in developing a translational research strategy to maximize the economic and health benefits of innovation'. It is essentially the key coordinating body and reports to the Department of Health and the Department for Innovation, Universities and Skills (DIUS), and plays a role in determining government health research strategy, bidding for funding from the Treasury and monitoring delivery of the strategy. In addition, it plays an important role in promoting a greater partnership between pharmaceutical and bioscience sectors, charities and government.

'What do you know about the Research Assessment Exercise?'

The Research Assessment Exercise (RAE) is an approximately 5 yearly national review of the quality of research produced by a higher education institution (HEI) conducted by the four higher education funding councils in the UK – the Higher Education Funding Council for England (HEFCE), the Scottish Funding Council (SFC), the Higher Education Funding Council for Wales (HEFCW) and the Department for Employment and Learning, Northern Ireland (DEL). HEI RAE submissions for each subject area (unit of assessment) are ranked by a specialist peer review panel and this will determine the research funding allocated to the institution by their national funding council. RAE 2008 is the sixth such exercise, with the main body of evidence being collected in 2007–2008 and outcomes published in December 2008.

RAE 2008 uses a four-point quality scale based on assessment of research outputs for each full-time member of staff, e.g., papers published, conference abstracts, etc., research environment as well as indicators of esteem, and generates a quality profile for each unit of assessment or subject area, e.g., medicine.

Following a *Review of Research Assessment* (Roberts Report 2003) the RAE (after 2008) is set to be replaced by a metrics-based approach using citation analysis – i.e., the number of research papers published and their impact as a method for allocating HEI funding.

A useful link to RAE 2008 can be found at www.rae.ac.uk.

Medical statistics

If you have performed or required statistical analysis of any of your work/research, then during the interview you should expect to be asked a little bit about the statistical methodologies that were used and why.

It is not the place of this book to go through medical statistics and we would strongly advise that you should either spend a short time talking with a medical statistician in preparation for your interview or reading around the subject in some of the short version books that are readily available.

Typical statistics-related questions

'What do you understand by the term randomized control trial (RCT)?'

- *Randomized control trial (RCT)*: A study in which people are allocated at random (by chance alone) to receive one of several clinical interventions. One of these interventions acts as a comparison to provide a benchmark. As the outcomes are measured, RCTs are quantitative studies. In addition, they may be single or double blinded.
- *Randomized*: Patients (subjects) are allocated a treatment option completely by chance using, for example, a random number generator.
- *Control*: Standard group against which the patients undergoing the experimental treatment option are compared.
- *Single blind*: Either the subject or the observers are unaware of which treatment option the subject has been assigned.
- *Double blind*: Both the subject and the observers are unaware of which treatment option the subject has been assigned.

'What is screening? (± Give examples of national screening programmes)'

'Screening is a public health service in which members of a defined population, who do not necessarily perceive they are at risk of, or are already affected by, a disease or its complications, are asked a question or offered a test to identify those individuals who are more likely to be helped than harmed by further tests or treatment to reduce the risk of a disease or its complications.' (UK National Screening Committee 2000)

The Wilson–Jungner criteria for appraising the validity of a screening programme, published by the World Health Organization in 1968, are outlined in Box 5.1.

Box 5.1

The Wilson–Jungner criteria for appraising the validity of a screening programme
1. The condition being screened for should be an important health problem
2. The natural history of the condition should be well understood
3. There should be a detectable early stage
4. Treatment at an early stage should be of more benefit than at a later stage
5. A suitable test should be devised for the early stage
6. The test should be acceptable
7. Intervals for repeating the test should be determined
8. Adequate health service provision should be made for the extra clinical workload resulting from screening
9. The risks, both physical and psychological, should be less than the benefits
10. The costs should be balanced against the benefits

After Wilson & Jungner (1968).

'What is meant by sensitivity and specificity?'

- *Sensitivity*: The proportion of subjects tested who have the disorder/disease and gain a positive result:

$$\text{Sensitivity} = \frac{\text{No. of true positives}}{\text{No. of true positives} + \text{No. of false negatives}}$$

- *Specificity*: The proportion of subjects tested who do not have the disorder/disease and gain a negative result:

$$\text{Specificity} = \frac{\text{No. of true negatives}}{\text{No. of true negatives} + \text{No. of false positives}}$$

(See also the Publications section in Further reading.)

Teaching

Teaching is often an important part of this section of the interview and you may be simply asked, 'Tell us what experience you have of teaching.' This question, although seemingly straightforward, requires preparation.

It is rather unimaginative when the trainee discusses his or her experience of teaching in terms of their undergraduate exposure and how they taught a senior group of trainees taking finals and how they all passed.

The approach you should take to this question is to acknowledge that you have experience of teaching undergraduates but then to discuss your experience of teaching postgraduates and where possible of assessing undergraduates. At this point you may even be able to talk about your involvement in the competency assessment of more junior trainees, which is a central part of Modernising Medical Careers (MMC) – for example, your involvement in the assessment of Foundation level trainees using mini-DOPs (directly observed procedures), mini-CEX (clinical evaluation exercises), 360-degree appraisal and case-based discussions.

It is also important in the teaching section to bring into the discussion any experience that you may have of teaching other healthcare professionals, remembering that there are others than just medical students – for instance, nurses, physiotherapists, ambulance crews, etc. Of course, if you have extensive teaching experience beyond those mentioned so far, e.g., experience of teaching, developing or organizing postgraduate and undergraduate courses, it is essential that you make sure that you discuss these in detail during the interview.

In addition, try to present some form of time commitment as to how often you teach and for how long. You may also be asked to 'describe your worst teaching experience' or to 'describe your best teaching experience'. You should prepare examples of both, appropriate to your own teaching strengths or weaknesses and your level of experience. It may be that the subject was too complicated for you and the audience were too advanced. It may have been an audience with a multi-disciplinary make-up. You may have learned the subject but not understood it adequately to be able to stand up to the questioning.

More generic questions about teaching may be, 'Why do you enjoy teaching?' or 'What makes a good teacher?' or 'What teaching methods do you prefer?'

Remember that teaching experience is not just about delivering teaching; it is also about how you have obtained your experience on teaching methodology. You may have attended various courses, e.g., 'Teaching the teachers', or have undertaken an intercalated medical education degree, and you should bring this into the discussion.

Further teaching-related questions

'How would you teach anatomy to surgeons in training?'

The 'dumbing-down' of anatomy teaching at medical school is a bugbear for many surgeons. Methods of bridging the gap in knowledge at postgraduate level are listed below, and experience or an appreciation of these is advantageous:

- Anatomy demonstrating/teaching; developing prosections
- Courses – with anatomy taught in the clinical context
- Assessment of anatomy within postgraduate examinations, e.g., MRCS
- Simulators; CD-ROM interactive packages
- Continuous assessment in daily practice by your consultant trainer.

'What is learning?'

This type of question does not merely intend for you to define your understanding of the term 'learning'; it is also a platform for you, having given a definition, to launch into a dialogue about your own experiences of teaching.

Questions similar to this will be used throughout your interview as a starter question and when preparing for the interview you should practise answering the question with the view to continuing the conversation in the direction that you want the interview to take – i.e., take control of the interview.

Learning can be defined as, 'the acquisition of knowledge or skill' or 'the knowledge or skill received by instruction or study' (Webster's Dictionary).

'What teaching formats are you aware of?'

There are a range of different teaching techniques and the type of teaching format you employ is determined by a number of factors including:

- The size of the group
- The level or age of the group, e.g., final year medical students, junior doctors
- The time allocated to teach
- The setting, e.g., theatre, clinic
- The subject matter or aim of teaching, e.g., practical skills, history.

Importantly, when answering this question you should aim to discuss the different techniques available in relation to your personal experience of them and the discussion may evolve to include the advantages and disadvantages of each.

Types of teaching formats include

- Lectures
- Seminars or tutorials: small or large group
- Bedside teaching
- Hands-on teaching, e.g., objective structured clinical examination (OSCE) skills
- Problem-based teaching/learning
- Role playing
- Demonstrations
- Case-based discussions
- Panel of experts
- Peer tutoring
- Simulators
- Computer-based learning.

'What factors make learning effective?'

Again, don't simply list the factors that make teaching/learning effective; relate them to your practice and experience.

For example: 'From my experience, I think there are a number of factors which play an important role … I think it's important to gauge the level of knowledge or first-hand experience of the topic the group has and this is also a useful way of engaging the class … In addition, right at the beginning I like to outline the aim and objectives I intend to cover … Also, especially when I do bedside small group teaching to medical students, I try to learn the students' names and this helps to facilitate a more interactive session and create a more relaxed environment.'

Factors required for effective teaching

- Adequate preparation
- Clearly defined aims and objectives – i.e., outcome driven
- Meaningful and purposeful content
- Teaching pitched at the appropriate level – i.e., establish prior knowledge
- Teaching based on the capacity to learn
- Active student participation
- Motivated students
- Allowing time for reflection and reinforcement of concepts
- Adequate feedback.

'What are the benefits or skills that you develop through teaching?'

The skills that you personally have acquired should be discussed in the context of the teaching that you have done to date. These skills may include:

- Confidence in public speaking
- Fluency with language
- Improved communication skills
- Ability to listen more effectively
- Self-reflection with identification of your personal strengths and weaknesses
- Responsibility
- More effective time management
- Leadership skills: ability to motivate others and drive learning
- Teamwork
- Interpersonal skills
- Ability to give and respond to feedback
- Improved IT skills, e.g., PowerPoint
- Awareness and use of resources available
- Ability to assimilate and present knowledge.

Associated questions

- How would you teach medical students? How would that differ from teaching a junior doctor?
- Tell me about your experiences in teaching.
- Which is more important – research or teaching?

Clinical governance, audit and management

This is the second section and may be replaced by a portfolio-based interview.

Clinical governance

Under this section, clinical governance will often be dealt with using clinical case scenarios, examples of which will be different for different specialities. An example in surgery may be, 'What do you do if a swab has been left in the wound and the nurse has acknowledged that her swab count is not correct at the end of the procedure.' Other similar clinical questions in surgery, may relate to the wrong side or site of operation or the general anaesthetic or the patient's identity. For example, 'The patient has come to the operating theatre without the operating site marked and the anaesthetist has put the patient to sleep before you realize it. How would you deal with this?' or 'How would you manage a situation where the identity of the patient under the anaesthetic has been called into question.'

In general medicine clinical scenarios may relate to your management of patients who have been given the wrong medication – either the wrong drug or the wrong dose – or have suffered a drug interaction.

It should be remembered that at the end of all of these clinical scenarios you should mention clinical incident reporting. If you mention clinical incident reporting you should then expect the question, 'What happens to the clinical incident form after you have completed it?' (see below).

Common clinical governance-related questions

What is clinical governance?

Clinical governance was introduced into the NHS following the Government's White Paper: *The New NHS: Modern, Dependable* (DH 1997).

> 'Clinical governance is the system through which NHS organizations are accountable for continuously improving the quality of their services and safeguarding high standards of care, by creating an environment in which clinical excellence will flourish.' (Sir Liam Donaldson, Chief Medical Officer, DH 1997)

There are 'seven pillars' (or components) which support the development of clinical governance (established by the National Clinical Governance Development Unit):

1. Clinical audit
2. Patient and public involvement
3. Clinical risk management
4. Clinical effectiveness
5. Staffing and staff management
6. Education and training, e.g., continuing professional development
7. Information used to facilitate the governance process.

'Who is responsible for clinical governance?'

All NHS bodies have a statutory duty and are accountable for continually improving the quality of their services and safeguarding standards of care.

- Within strategic health authorities (SHAs) the Clinical Governance League is responsible for ensuring there is a clinical audit programme within local trusts and that this reflects national audit priorities.
- The chief executive and medical director are responsible for the quality of care delivered by the organization. The chief executive and/or medical

director may choose to appoint a clinical governance lead (not necessarily a clinician) to assist with the coordination of governance activity, e.g., audits within the organization.

'What is the process of clinical governance?'

For clinical governance to be successful there are a number of fundamental requirements, namely:

- Teamwork
- A commitment to the aims of clinical governance
- Good communication
- Ownership of the ideas
- Leadership
- Systems awareness.

The 'RAID' model is a well-established mechanism for implementing change:

R – Review: gather information and assess 'where you are at'
A – Agree: gain a consensus, establish teams and formulate recommendations
I – Implement: requires project management, prioritization and motivation of supporting staff
D – Demonstrate: involves project analysis, identifying lessons learnt and planning the next objective.

'What do you understand by the term clinical effectiveness?'

Clinical effectiveness is 'the extent to which specific clinical interventions (e.g. a treatment, procedure or service) when deployed in the field for a particular patient or population do what they are intended to do, that is, maintain and improve health and secure the greatest possible health gain from the available resources' (NHS Executive 1996). More simply, clinical effectiveness is 'doing the right thing the right way at the right time' (Kibbe et al. 1994). In order for clinical effectiveness to be successful, all healthcare professionals need to be able to readily access information regarding best practice and evidence-based approaches and this information must be reliable and comprehensive.

Clinical effectiveness has three key components:

1. *Obtaining the evidence*: This is predominantly acquired and collated from research studies, e.g., randomized control trials and systematic reviews.
2. *Implementation*: Changing practice in light of the evidence – i.e. 'evidence-based practice'. This can be achieved by the use of national standards, e.g.,

the national service frameworks (NSFs) or national clinical guidelines, e.g., NICE guidelines, and requires the dissemination of information as well as the availability of resources to support practice.

3. *Evaluation* of the impact of practice and adaptation – i.e., assessment of clinical outcome, usually in the context of a clinical audit with changes in practice and re-audit.

Note: You may be asked to give an example where you have applied research-based evidence in clinical practice with a resulting improvement in patient outcome, e.g., statin therapy for the secondary prevention of stroke as recommended following the SPARCL trial and the Heart Protection Study.

'What is clinical risk management?'

Clinical risk management (CRM) forms part of *The NHS Plan* (2000a) and is the systematic approach to improving the safety and quality of healthcare (both clinical and non-clinical) delivered in the NHS by identifying and assessing, as well as analyzing and prioritizing, the risk to patients, staff and members of the public and acting to prevent or control them, e.g., by redesigning systems/structures to reduce human error and developing improvement strategies.

Clinical risk can be assessed through:

- Critical incident reporting of adverse clinical events or 'near misses'
- Screening or auditing patient medical records.

A useful link to the Department of Health clinical governance website can be found at www.dh.gov.uk/en/Policyandguidance/Healthandsocialcaretopics/Clinicalgovernance/index.htm

'How do you reduce the risk of hospital-acquired infections?'

Infection control is a very emotive topic and it would be unusual for you not to have come across issues surrounding infection control or 'outbreaks' in your practice to date. You should try to answer this question in relation to your experiences and your current hospital's infection control policy – which you should be able to download from your hospital intranet site.

Healthcare associated infections (HCAIs) are infections transmitted to patients (and healthcare workers) as a result of healthcare procedures, in hospital and other healthcare settings. An estimated 9% of inpatients have an HCAI at any one time and the Office of National Statistics put the number of deaths from MRSA at 51 in 1993 and 955 in 2003.

The most commonly implicated pathogens are meticillin-resistant *Staphylococcus aureus* (MRSA), vancomycin-resistant *Staphylococcus aureus* (VRSA), *Escherichia coli* (*E. coli*), *Pseudomonas aeruginosa* (*P. aeruginosa*), *Klebsiella pneumoniae* (*K. pneumoniae*), glycopeptide-resistant enterococci (GRE) and *Clostridium difficile* (*C. difficile*).

Strategies to reduce infection require the education and cooperation of all staff, patients and visitors. Most hospitals will have an Infection Control Team which plays a central role in advising on infection control measures as well as auditing hospital infection rates for 'outbreaks' and monitoring compliance to existing infection control strategies. These strategies may include:

Changes to the hospital environment

- The use of side rooms rather than open wards
- Separate isolation floors or wards for patients with infections, e.g., *C. difficile* with designated nursing staff
- Ample access to wash basins and alcohol gel
- Laminar air flow systems (typically used in orthopaedic and cardiothoracic theatres)
- Easy-to-clean computer stations
- Sloping surfaces (desk tops and floors) that do not accumulate dust
- Reduced bed occupancy rates (currently within the NHS it is >82%)
- Greater investment in infection control
- Mandatory surveillance of HCAIs within hospitals; this came into effect for MRSA in 2001 and for GRE and *C. difficile* in 2003 and 2004, respectively
- More evidence-based research on prevention of HCAIs (of which there is a paucity).

Behavioural changes – development of a 'culture of cleanliness'

It is estimated that between 15 and 30% of HCAIs could be prevented by better hygiene practices. Changes to hygiene practices may be broadly described as being 'patient-centred' or 'staff-centred'.

- Patient-centred changes
  - Education in infection control
  - Screening for infections, e.g., MRSA pre-admission (MRSA colonization can be up to 5%) and prior to interhospital transfer
  - Treatment of infections, e.g., oral metronidazole for *C. difficile* infection
  - Requesting visitors and staff to wash hands
  - Reporting of areas which are not clean, e.g., bathrooms
  - Prophylactic chlorhexidine washes preceding surgery.

- Staff-centred changes
  - ○ Education in infection control and good communication
  - ○ Reporting of areas which are not clean
  - ○ Meticulous hand washing/alcohol gel use
  - ○ Use of appropriate barriers, e.g., gloves, aprons, face masks and glasses
  - ○ Disposal of sharps and clinical waste appropriately
  - ○ Appropriate management of spillages of blood or bodily fluids
  - ○ Adequate decontamination of equipment, e.g., clean, disinfect or desterilize as appropriate to the level of contamination
  - ○ Avoidance of indiscriminate or prolonged use of antibiotics, e.g., cephalosporins; microbiology advice as appropriate
  - ○ Use of antibiotic prophylaxis may reduce the risk of infection perioperatively (at induction) or for invasive procedures, e.g., urinary catheterization, as appropriate.

(See also the Clinical governance section in Further reading.)

'What do you understand by the term critical incidence reporting?'

It should be remembered that the final point of any discussion related to issues of clinical governance is critical incidence reporting and often in this part the interviewer is interested to know whether you understand critical incidence reporting, what happens to the forms after they have been completed, what feedback is given as a result of a clinical incident, and how it is determined whether the event is an isolated incident or whether it conforms with a pattern.

Critical incidence forms require you to record the following:

- Date of the event – this should be as soon after the event as possible
- Reporting team member
- Date, time and location of the incident
- Team members involved
- Description of incident – this should be balanced and factual
- How the situation was managed and the outcome.

In most trusts this form will eventually go to the quality assurance committee who will look at it to see whether this is a one-off incident and whether there is anything that can be learnt from it, or whether it is part of a pattern of behaviour that may need to be looked at in more detail. The objective of the clinical incident reporting system is to make the service better and everyone in the service should be encourage to complete these forms. It is not designed as a mechanism for punishing people.

'What is the role of the National Patient Safety Agency?'

The National Patient Safety Agency (NPSA) aims to put patient safety at the top of the NHS agenda and encourages greater transparency and accountability promoting a culture of no-blame within the NHS for the provision of safer healthcare.

The NPSA includes a patient safety division which collects, analyzes and prioritizes data on adverse incidents involving patients in the NHS; where risks are identified, the NPSA ensures work is undertaken to produce solutions to prevent these accidents and incidents recurring.

Importantly, the NPSA oversees three independent confidential enquiries: National Confidential Enquiry into Patient Outcome and Death (NCEPOD), Confidential Enquiry into Suicide and Homicides (CESH) and Confidential Enquiry into Maternal and Child Health (CEMACH). These enquiries draw on evidence on all hospital activity within the UK and include data from the Defence Sector, NHS and private sectors. The aim of this data collection is to monitor and subsequently improve upon the quality and safety of patient care delivered.

In addition, the NPSA is also responsible for supporting local organizations in addressing their concerns about the performance of individual doctors and dentists, safety aspects of hospital design, hospital cleanliness, food standards and for ensuring clinical research is carried out safely and ethically.

Another obvious and very clear example of the work of the NPSA is the presence of the lay-chairman at the medical interviews. Most committees within the NHS will have lay representation.

Further clinical governance-related questions

- How does clinical governance affect your daily practice?
- Is clinical governance necessary?
- What do you understand by clinical governance? Discuss one component, giving an example.
- A patient who has a penicillin allergy is accidentally administered penicillin. How would you tackle this?
- Tell me about a mistake that you've made.
- How do you explain to a patient that the wrong side has been operated on?
- Give an example where the outcome of an action you took in response to a clinical mistake/error made you reassess how you would deal with a similar events in the future.

Audit

Audit should have been conducted by everybody undertaking an interview at this stage. Audit questions will usually start along the lines of, 'Discuss one of the audits that you have done.' or 'Tell me about your most interesting audit.' or 'Tell me about the audit that you think is the most valuable.'

You will be expected to discuss an audit(s) that you have undertaken, why you undertook them, what results you obtained and, of course, what has been done to close the loop and the impact of the audit on your clinical practice.

In the vast majority of instances trainees will talk about the first part and then will use the fact that they have rotated on to another job as an excuse for the audit-loop not being closed. It is far more appropriate, if a proper audit has been performed and a problem identified that can be corrected, that the correction is put in place and the next trainee coming in should re-audit it at a later date. The handling of the question should reflect this, and you should discuss the changes that should be enforced before the audit cycle is completed unless that process is not being planned. Differences between audit and research must be understood, as well as the purpose of performing audit.

Common audit-related questions

'What is audit?'

Audit is an evaluation of a person, organization, system process project or product and is used to ascertain the validity and reliability of information as well as acting as a system of internal control.

'What is clinical audit?'

'Clinical audit is a quality improvement process that seeks to improve patient care and outcomes through systematic review of care against explicit criteria and implementation of change. Aspects of the structure, processes and outcomes of care are selected and systematically evaluated against explicit criteria. Where indicated, changes are implemented at an individual, team or service level and further monitoring is used to confirm improvement in healthcare delivery.' (NICE & Healthcare Commission 2002).

Components of the Audit Cycle

- Setting standards
- Measuring current practice
- Comparing results with standards
- Changing practice
- Re-auditing to ensure practice improves i.e. completing the audit cycle

---

'What are the benefits of audit?'

The main purpose of an audit is to increase the quality of service (i.e., it is a key component of clinical governance). In addition, it helps to identify and promote good clinical practice (i.e., evidence-based practice) and also ensures that the outcomes are in line with peer practice, both within the hospital and nationally.

'How does audit differ from research?'

Be prepared for the question asking about the differences between research and audit.

'Research is concerned with discovering the right thing to do; audit is ensuring that it is done right' (Smith 1992).

Similarities between audit and research

- Both start with a question relating to quality of care
- Both produce results which intend to change practice
- Both can be carried out retrospectively or prospectively
- Both involve developing a methodology, data collection, sampling and analysis of findings with conclusions.

Differences between research and audit

- Audit, unlike research
  - Assesses current practice against a standard which is determined by research and aims to identify ways in which the service can be improved specific to the group being studied and is practice based
  - Is a continuous process and involves changes to practice and then re-auditing.
- Research, unlike audit
  - Creates new knowledge, thus increasing the amount of knowledge already in existence
  - Requires ethical approval – i.e., referral to the Research Ethics Committee (REC)
  - May involve random allocation to different treatment groups ± a placebo group
  - Produces results which may be applied to clinical practice globally rather than limited to local practice
  - Identifies areas for auditing (can be vice versa)
  - Is not a continuous process but is a one-off study.

'How do you ensure that you improve the quality of care you deliver to your patients?'

This is a question that centres on audit and clinical governance and would ideally be answered by giving an example of an audit that you have performed with a discussion of any changes implemented and whether a re-audit was performed to complete the 'audit cycle'.

'What is the National Audit Office?'

The National Audit Office (NAO)/Audit Commission is an independent organization that scrutinizes public spending on behalf of parliament and is responsible for ensuring that public money is spent economically, efficiently and effectively to achieve high quality local services to the public.

'What is research governance?'

Research governance can be defined as the broad range of regulations, principles and standards of good practice that exist to achieve, and continuously improve, research quality across all aspects of healthcare in the UK and worldwide (Clinical Research Governance Office, Imperial College, London).

The Department of Health requires anyone undertaking research within an NHS trust or medical school to adhere to the rules set out in *The Research Governance Framework for Health and Social Care* (DH 2005), namely that all researchers carrying out clinically oriented research within the trust:

- Must possess a trust substantive or honorary contract
- Must obtain approval of the R&D directorate and the appropriate research ethics committee before any research commences
- Have a responsibility for the conduct of their research and must ensure that any research follows the agreed protocol and complies with all the legal and ethical requirements throughout the course of the research
- Must comply with research monitoring and audit as required and provide reports on progress and outcomes if requested by the trust or financial sponsors
- Must make available findings from their research promptly and feed this back to participants if appropriate or requested
- Have a responsibility for the management of the financial and other resources including the management of any intellectual property rights, in relation to their research.

Further audit-related questions

- Which of your research or audit studies has made the greatest contribution to your practice and why? What was your level of involvement and the outcome?

For a useful link, see the Audit Commission website (www.audit-commission.gov.uk); see also the Audit section in Further reading.

Management

Management for junior trainees is a much more difficult topic to discuss at interview, probably because most have had little experience of it at this stage. During discussions on management it is far more likely that the panel will be talking about specific areas such as NICE, the European Working Time Directive (EWTD), MMC, etc. The key topics, you should at least be aware of, will be outlined in the remainder of this chapter.

National Institute for Health and Clinical Excellence

All trainees should know about the National Institute for Health and Clinical Excellence (NICE).

NICE is 'an independent organization responsible for developing national guidance on the promotion of good health and the prevention and treatment of ill health'. NICE was established in 1999, following the White Paper *A First Class Service* (DH 1998) and the NHS is legally obliged to provide funding and resources in England and Wales for medicines and treatments recommended by NICE's technology appraisal guidance.

Guidelines are produced in three key areas:

1. *Public health*: The promotion of good health and the prevention of ill health, e.g., smoking in the workplace.
2. *Health technology*: The use of new and existing drugs, medical devices, e.g., inhalers, diagnostic techniques, surgical procedures and health promotion activities within the NHS.
3. *Clinical practice*: The appropriate treatment and care of patients with specific diseases and conditions. This covers diagnosis, treatment, care and self-help.

Guidelines which fulfil the requirements of evidence-based practice are established by an independent group of experts following extensive consultation (i.e., NICE's appraisal committee), with evidence collated from a number of sources:

- Good quality studies
- Knowledge from doctors' and specialists' knowledge
- Knowledge from individuals with specialist knowledge, e.g., organizations representing the views of patients.

Occasionally, an individual practitioner's approach to managing a condition over many years may have produced excellent results but differs from the general advice given by NICE. In these instances, provided the practitioner's approach to the condition produces results that are acceptable when compared to their peer groups, then that clinician will not have to alter their clinical practice. For the majority of people in clinical practice, however, the NICE guidelines will need to be utilized.

Controversies with NICE

NICE can produce conflicting advice. For instance, the rationing of drugs has previously been recommended on the basis of cost and, as a result, a drug may be available on the NHS in some parts of the country but not in others.

Associated question

- Describe one NICE guideline in relation to your speciality.

For a useful link, see the NICE website (www.nice.org.uk); see also the Management section in Further reading.

The European Working Time Directive (EWTD)

The European Working Time Directive is European Union (EU) health and safety legislation, which dictates the number of hours you can work as well as how much rest you should take. Adherence to the directive is not optional. Working time includes any period during which you are working, including any period during which you are receiving relevant training. Although you will not be expected to know all the regulations, the important aspects you should be aware of are that:

- By 2009, the total average maximum number of hours worked (including educational time) should not exceed 48 hours per week
- The EWTD also advises on rest and break requirements and states that there must be:
  - A minimum of 11 hours continuous rest in every 24-hour period
  - A minimum period of 24 hours' continuous rest in every 7-day period worked

○ A minimum break of 20 minutes after every 6 hours worked
○ A minimum of 4 weeks' paid annual leave
○ A maximum of 8 hours' work in each 24 hours for night workers.

In addition to the EWTD, you should be aware of two further rulings (which pertain to the interpretation of the Working Time Directive) which have had a major impact on the work patterns of doctors, namely:

- The *SiMAP* case in which the European Court of Justice ruled that:
  ○ Time spent on-call must be regarded in its entirety as 'working time' within the meaning of the Directive
  ○ If one merely had to be contactable at all times when on-call (i.e., non-resident), only time linked to the actual provision of primary healthcare services should be regarded as 'working time'
  ○ In both the above scenarios, compensatory rest must be factored in before the next period of work.
- The *Jaeger* case in which the European Court of Justice ruled that:
  ○ On-call duty performed by a doctor where he is required to be physically present in the hospital must be regarded as working time in its totality (as above)
  ○ Periods when a doctor is *resident* on-call but not working, e.g., resting or asleep, should *not* be regarded as rest periods
  ○ If 11 hours' continuous rest is not achieved in each 24-hour period, then compensation (time) must be given.

Any discussions on the EWTD are likely to naturally lead on to questions on rotas, shift-working and schemes such as Hospital at Night.

Common EWTD-related questions

'What is the likely impact of the EWTD on training and how can this be minimized?'

At interview the obvious difficult area relates to how one trains, particularly those trainees in craft specialities, such as surgery and obstetrics and gynaecology, within the constraints of the hours imposed by the EWTD. It is likely that training will be more streamlined and that, probably, as time moves forward, educationally numbered posts will in the majority be supernumerary. This is not in place at the present moment but as MMC progresses this will undoubtedly be an inevitable outcome.

In summary, with the reduction in hours, there will be less time available to train and in order to train to CCT level:

- Training will need to be competency-based rather than time-based

- Total time spent in training may need to be lengthened
- Fellowships (i.e., a period of time spent at the end of training within a specialist centre to improve specific skills, e.g., interventional or laparoscopic) are likely to become commonplace
- The product of training will be a specialist rather than the old-school generalist
- Tasks not necessarily required to be performed by doctors, as already the case with phlebotomy, will need to be taken on by other allied healthcare professionals
- Training posts may in the future become supernumerary with a greater proportion of training under consultant supervision – i.e., the trainee is there almost exclusively to be trained
- Elective and emergency commitments must be separated for both the trainer and trainee in order to maximize daytime educational opportunities.

The benefit of the EWTD is better work–life balance.

'How can you maximize training opportunities with the EWTD?'

- Rota design
  - Organizing trainees' time around training opportunities – i.e., design the rota which will maximize the training activities within your hospital. It may be appropriate for more senior colleagues to be non-resident on-call or removed from the night-shift rota to maximize daytime training opportunities
  - Separating elective and emergency commitments for both trainer and trainee
  - Recognizing educational activity as an integral part of the week
  - Factoring education into your trainer's job plan
- Dedicated training (rather than service) lists and the use of parallel lists
- Establishment of training units/centres
- Avoidance of conflicts of training opportunities with fellow trainees, e.g., through pairing of more junior with more senior trainees who will need to acquire different competencies
- The use of virtual reality simulators
- Regular appraisal and development of an educational plan with goal setting.

'What is the likely impact of EWTD on patterns of working?'

- With a reduction in hours, there will be the inevitable change from on-call to shift patterns of working.

- Continuity of patient care will only be possible with adequate handover processes in place.
- There will need to be a delegation of responsibilities to other professionals, e.g., nurse consultants and the development of Hospital at Night-type working practices.

Consultants and the EWTD

Currently, consultants within the NHS have been able to opt out of the EWTD, but in 2009 they will need to be compliant with the 48 hours initiative. It would seem very difficult for this to be reached, certainly without a massive expansion in consultant numbers, and the implementation of EWTD compliance to the consultant grade may well be deferred.

Subspecialization

'What do you think about increasing subspecialization?'

Subspecialization is inevitable in the current training climate and when answering this question you should be able to demonstrate a clear understanding of the advantages and disadvantages, especially in terms of training.

Advantages of subspecialization

- Concentrated expertise in a particular area resulting in improved quality of patient care, e.g., reduced operative mortality, reduced operating times
- A reduction in the overall cost of delivery of healthcare
- Improved training within a subspeciality within a specialist centre
- Greater progress in the development of diagnostic tools and treatments due to pooled expertise within a field
- Improved and more coordinated research
- The subspecialist may be a more achievable endpoint within the constraints of the EWTD.

Disadvantages of subspecialization

- A greater number of referrals to specialist teams previously managed by more general medical or surgical teams
- Lack of appropriate funding to fund subspeciality training
- Skills are less transportable globally
- Need to decide on speciality at an earlier stage in your career
- Lower standards of care for those unable to access subspeciality services
- Inability of individual doctors to deal with a patient with a complexity of multiple pathology.

Associated questions

- Do you think you will be ready in 5 years to take on a consultant post?
- How would you design a rota to ensure your training needs were met under the EWTD?

MMC

Modernising Medical Careers sets out the principles underpinning the long-awaited reform of postgraduate medical education and training and is a concept that takes roots from Sir Liam Donaldson's paper *Unfinished Business* (DH 2002a).

In essence, MMC proposes (DH 2004a):

- Competitive, UK-wide entry into an integrated, seamless and planned 2-year Foundation programme of general training, which is:
  - Structured
  - Trainee-centred
  - Outcome based and competency assessed, with robust methods of assessment
  - Quality assured

  with the first year equating to the current pre-registration house officer year and the second year incorporating a broad-based, generic first year of current SHO training
- Following the Foundation programme, open competitive entry into run-through specialist and general practice training
- Once accepted into run-through training, seamless, competency-based progression to CCT.

  In addition there will be:
- An exit route from specialist training programmes into what are now termed the non-consultant career grades
- Opportunities to change direction
- Constructive careers advice linked with mentoring, coaching and counselling systems.

The allocation of numbered training posts into the run-through system should reflect workforce requirements and will be determined by the MMC Board, which includes representatives from the BMA, Academy of Medical Royal Colleges and NHS. The task of defining the principles and standards which form the basis of assessment and approving Foundation programme posts is charged to the Postgraduate Medical Education and Training Board (PMETB).

The original principles underlying MMC were a subject under review in the Tooke Report (see below).

Common MMC-related questions

'What do you understand by the term competence?'

Competence is 'the possession of requisite or adequate ability, having acquired the knowledge and skills necessary to perform those tasks which reflect the scope of professional practices. It may be different from *performance,* which denotes what someone is actually doing in a real life situation.'

Competencies are a set of observed behaviours and 'professional abilities that includes elements of knowledge, skills, attitudes and experience' (PMETB 2005).

Associated questions

- What do you think of competency-based training?
- What are the disadvantages of evaluating Foundation year doctors?

The Tooke Report

As a result of the problems encountered with the Medical Training Application Service (MTAS) during the recruitment process into specialist training in 2007, a national enquiry led by Professor Sir John Tooke, called the Tooke Report, was undertaken. This reported in January 2008.

In general the Report has received widespread support from all sectors of the medical profession and identifies eight key areas for action (adapted from the Tooke Report; MMC Inquiry 2008):

1. Clarification of the objectives of postgraduate medical training and the development of mechanisms to achieve these
2. Clarification of the role of doctors at different stages in their career
3. Strengthening of DH policy on development and alignment implementation and governance
4. Workforce planning – in particular to address the 'bulge' at SHO level
5. Strengthening of the medical profession's ability to influence health policy
6. Strengthening of the commissioning and management of postgraduate medical training
7. Streamlining of the regulation of medical education
8. Adaptation of the structure of postgraduate medical education and training (PMET) to meet the principles underpinning Modernising Medical Careers, e.g., flexibility, broad-based beginnings and an aspiration to excellence.

The final report makes 47 recommendations regarding both speciality training and the appointments process; however, it is unclear how many of these will be adopted in the future.

Although you are not expected to know all of the recommendations, there are some that you should be aware of, namely:

- Formation of a new body to oversee postgraduate medical education and training – NHS: Medical Education England (NHS: MEE)
- Active exploration of ways of legally offsetting or compensating for the EWTD, which has been detrimental to PMET
- Uncoupling of the Foundation year and abandonment of run-through training – i.e., a single pre-registration year, followed by 3 core years specialist training
- Shortlisting for interview to entry to higher specialist training to include formal assessments by national assessment centres
- Completion of higher speciality training to lead to a Certificate of Completion of Training (CCT)
- Length of training for GPs to be extended to 5 years (3 core years training + 2 years in specialist registrar training)
- Merging of PMETB with the GMC to 'facilitate a common philosophy and approach across the continuum of medical education … with the sharing of quality enhancement expertise'.

Postgraduate Medical Education and Training Board (PMETB)

Established in 2003, the Postgraduate Medical Education and Training Board (www.pmetb.org.uk) is the independent regulatory body responsible for setting standards in postgraduate medical education and training. It takes over these responsibilities from the Specialist Training Authority of the Medical Royal Colleges and the Joint Committee on Postgraduate General Practice Training.

PMETB's vision is 'to achieve excellence in postgraduate medical education, training, assessment and accreditation throughout the UK to improve the knowledge, skills and experience of doctors and the health and healthcare of patients and the public' (PMETB 2008) and it achieves this vision through:

- Quality assuring training programmes and posts and monitoring training and training outcomes
- Defining the standards for selection into specialist selection
- Approving specialist curricula and assessments

- Maintaining standards for and certifying doctors for entry to the specialist and GP registers
- Independently leading policy development for the future of postgraduate medical education and training.

Workforce planning

'What do you understand by the term workforce planning?'

The aim of workforce planning is to produce, through our training programmes (i.e., through regulating the number of medical students trained and specialist training posts available), the right number of consultants and GPs per year to meet the service delivery requirements within the NHS. In theory, if workforce planning is successful, the number of consultants and GPs completing training should match the posts available.

Predicting the make-up of and planning the future workforce is exceptionally difficult, not least because training programmes for speciality training often last 8 years and the requirements and needs of the workforce within the NHS often change in cycles which are less than that.

Currently, there are more people coming out at the top end, having completed their training programmes, than there are posts for them to be appointed to – this is due not necessarily to a failing in workforce planning, but to cost.

The implementation of the EWTD, as well as the greater involvement of senior doctors in management, governance committees, research and education, means there is undoubtedly a need for massive consultant expansion in order to run the service as well as to train junior doctors for the future. However, this required expansion has been stunted due to the financial crisis within the NHS, which can therefore be seen to quite clearly and unpredictably impact on workforce planning.

Summary of factors affecting workforce planning (HM Treasury 2002)

- Resource/financial constraints
- Greater desire to train flexibly (i.e., work–life balance), an increasingly important consideration as a greater proportion of doctors in the future will be female
- Increasing non-clinical workload at consultant level, e.g., management, teaching
- Service requirements affected by system reform, e.g., greater drive towards care in the community
- Greater skill mix – i.e., more duties previous undertaken by doctors, now provided by other health professionals

- Poor retention of doctors
- Increasing student debt – less incentive to train as a doctor.

Hospital at Night (H@N)

The Hospital at Night scheme is an initiative spearheaded by Dr Elisabeth Paice, the then Dean Director for London, which aims to 'achieve effective clinical care at night by having one or more multi-disciplinary teams working in the hospital, who between them have the full range of skills and competencies to meet the patient's immediate needs' (NHS Modernisation Agency 2004).

In essence, Hospital at Night has 'redefined how medical cover is provided in hospitals during the out of hours period' with cover being defined by competencies. By taking this approach, a significant number of doctors may then be released from working night-time shifts or made non-resident on-call, thus supporting compliance with EWTD and enhancing training by increasing availability for programmed daytime activities.

Summary of the key principles of Hospital at Night

- Team working – each member has a defined role
- Multi-disciplinary and competency-based approach
- Extended nurse roles to perform jobs such as catheterization, venesection, etc. previously undertaken by doctors
- Skilled nurses to act as clinical coordinators to assess patients and contact the appropriate member of the team
- Effective bleep systems
- Improved handover arrangements
- Use of existing technologies to support the scheme, e.g., picture archiving and communications systems (PACS) available at home.

Advantages of Hospital at Night

- Improved quality of care reflected by shorter length of hospital stay
- Improved communication
- Better coordinated care
- Improved risk assessment and prioritization of care
- Reduced duplication of work, e.g., multiple clerking.

Disadvantages of Hospital at Night

- Cost implications often prevent full implementation of the scheme

- Perceived threat to tasks traditionally performed by doctors
- Potential impact on medical training
- A skeleton medical crew only is available at night
- Failure of change of the working pattern of other staff to support the scheme, e.g., extended hours beyond 5 pm for administrative staff to cover the busiest period for admission
- Inadequate recruitment and training of nurse coordinators to support the scheme
- Doctors may be required to cross-cover specialities, e.g., plastic surgery and orthopaedic surgery or cardiology and cardiothoracic surgery.

Common H@N-related questions

'What is the role of independent care practitioners?'

Independent care practitioners are generally nurses (but can be non-medical), working in clinical practice, who have been trained to a certain level to perform specific duties that traditionally were undertaken by doctors. Due to their very specific training and very carefully defined parameters of practice, the role of independent care practitioners within the NHS is essentially for service provision only. Examples include emergency nurse practitioners, emergency minor illnesses practitioners, nurses undertaking cystoscopy and sigmoidoscopy, nurses harvesting veins for coronary artery bypass grafting (CABG). Examples should be sought from the speciality relevant to the trainee.

Further question

- What are the main controversies surrounding independent care practitioners or surgical care practitioners?

Other important areas within this section

Other important topics on management can be categorized for the purpose of revision into 3 broad areas – Regulation of the Medical Profession, Management within the NHS and NHS Initiatives and Reforms. Common topics within these areas are discussed below.

Regulation of the medical profession

There have been many changes made to the General Medical Council recently, especially in relation to medical regulation and registration and you should be aware of these for the interview.

In the past, practitioners were given provisional registration and required to satisfactorily complete a period of 1 year as a pre-registration house officer (PRHO) in acute medicine and acute surgery, before achieving full registration. With MMC, the PRHO year has been superseded by a 2-year Foundation school programme. During the first year of Foundation training (FY1), practitioners who can demonstrate that they have achieved the relevant generic competencies can become fully registered at the end of FY1.

The regulations regarding the requirements that need to be achieved during the first year following graduation have, however, been considerably relaxed, and almost any programme of medical training is currently acceptable during the first year.

Common questions related to medical regulation

'What is appraisal?'

Appraisal is a broad topic for discussion and you may be simply asked, 'What is an appraisal?' or 'What is the objective of an appraisal?'

Appraisal is a positive forward-looking process, which gives doctors being appraised (the appraisee) the opportunity to reflect on their medical practice and to discuss areas for improvement, to receive feedback on past performance and to identify their individual educational and clinical development requirements. Evidence of annual appraisal within a managed organization with appropriate documentation is needed to fulfil the requirements of revalidation.

'How does assessment differ from appraisal? How would you assess a trainee?'

Assessment is a formal process which measures achievement and progress. It can be summative (i.e., contribute towards an endpoint) or formative. In medicine, a number of assessment tools or methods are utilized to assess all areas of *Good Medical Practice* (see Chapter 1). Appraisal, in contrast, is a mutual review by appraiser and appraisee of performance and progress, which results in identification of learning/training needs and goal setting.

'What is revalidation?'

The aim of revalidation is to protect patients from poorly performing doctors, promote good medical practice and increase public confidence in doctors.

Revalidation requires doctors to demonstrate their fitness to practise on a regular basis, every 3–5 years, and follows Dame Janet Smith's enquiry into the Shipman affair, the report of which was highly critical of the GMC.

As part of the process of revalidation, doctors will undergo revalidation by, first of all, relicensing on an annual basis and, for those on the specialist and GP registers, there would be a recertification process approximately every 5 years. This process would take into consideration the annual appraisals and doctors will need to demonstrate that they meet the standards set by the relevant Royal College and specialist association.

In 2006, Sir Liam Donaldson, the Chief Medical Officer, published his review into the regulation of the medical profession called *Good Doctors, Safer Patients* (DH 2006a). This recommended devolution of power of the GMC by having accredited GMC affiliates, greater public/patient involvement in decision making around fitness to practise and in the process of recertification.

In addition, the review recommends changes to professional regulation and requires regulatory bodies to use the civil standard, rather than the criminal standard, of proof when investigating fitness to practise, with a renewed focus on the assessment, rehabilitation and supervision of doctors with performance problems. Where these problems are not borne of malice there would be the creation of unambiguous standards, generic and specialist practice. These standards would be incorporated into the contracts of doctors.

'What is continuing professional development'?

'Continuing professional development (CPD) is a continuing learning process that complements formal undergraduate and postgraduate education and training. CPD requires doctors to maintain and improve their standards across all areas of their practice … CPD should also encourage and support specific changes in practice and career development. It has a role to play in helping doctors to keep up to date when they are not practising.' (GMC 2006a)

Management within the NHS

'What is the role of the clinical director?'

The clinical director is a consultant, appointed by the trust, responsible for service delivery within or across a number of specialities. He/she reports directly to the chief executive and is supported in this role by nurse and business managers and other senior clinical staff.

Clinical directors have executive power, authority and accountability for planning and developing services and the use of resources within their directorate and thus are responsible for:

● Providing the necessary clinical input for resource allocation

- Managing and planning service delivery
- Identifying service development priorities
- Development and execution of a business plan for the directorate
- Developing and negotiating annual budgets
- Establishing, developing and implementing clinical audit in the context of clinical governance
- Promoting and developing clinical outcome measures, monitoring directorate and individual performance and addressing underperformance
- Implementing risk management policies and monitoring as well as ensuring compliance
- Assessing performance of the directorate against targets
- Implementing the grievance/disciplinary process
- Ensuring a consistent approach across the directorate to standards/clinical protocols
- Ensuring effective communications within the directorate, in particular in relation to the dissemination of clinical information
- Supporting continuing professional development
- Recruiting medical staff (both temporary and permanent).

'What is the role of the chief executive of an NHS trust?'

The chief executive is the organizational head, spokesperson and leader of the NHS trust and is responsible for both the financial and managerial performance of their unit. In addition, they are also responsible for the quality of clinical care delivery, a role which they share with clinicians through the process of clinical governance. The role of chief executive within the NHS was created in the 1990s and is a role that is still relatively new and evolving.

The chief executive reports to the trust board which is composed of executive and non-executive directors (the majority) and who are ultimately accountable to the public and government. In summary, chief executives are responsible for:

- The financial and managerial performance of their organization, e.g., achievement of targets
- The quality of clinical care delivered and therefore clinical governance
- Implementation of new governmental policy, e.g., *The NHS Plan* (DH 2000a)
- Establishing collaborations outside the trust to ensure national policy is implemented, e.g., cancer networks
- Initiating and developing projects which may involve collaborating or negotiating with the private sector in private finance initiatives or through the contracting out of services

- Motivating the workforce and nurturing cultural change, as required
- Putting into place systems including resources and research, training and development opportunities, to ensure clinical standards are achieved
- Monitoring clinical standards and performance and, where they fall short, implementing changes to redress the balance
- Disseminating information within and outside the NHS organization.

A good relationship between the chief executive and the medical director is crucial for the success of clinical governance.

'What are managed clinical networks?'

Managed clinical networks (MCNs) are defined as: 'linked groups of health professionals and organizations from primary, secondary and tertiary care, working in a coordinated manner, unconstrained by existing professional and Health Board boundaries, to ensure equitable provision of high quality clinically effective services'. (NHS Management Executive 1999)

Networks can relate to a specific disease (e.g., diabetes, stroke, coronary heart disease, cancer), a speciality (e.g., neurology, vascular surgery) or a specific service (e.g., diagnostic services, pathology, accident and emergency) and may be local, regional or national (i.e., where the disease or service is rare or specialized).

Advantages of MCNs and centralization of services

- More equitably delivers to healthcare
- Vulnerable services which may have been 'lost' due to a shortage of expertise with increasing subspecialization and reduced hours of work (with EWTD) are maintained
- Care is standardized
- Information is shared across the network, thus resources are not duplicated
- Greater coordination and streamlining of the patient care pathway
- Waiting times may be improved
- Quality of care is improved due to access to an increased range of subspecialities within the network
- Resources including the workforce are more efficiently utilized
- Multi-disciplinary and multi-professional team working is encouraged
- Easier to train and maintain skills due to a higher exposure to relevant cases
- Discourages low volume operators (the recommendation from NICE is that surgeons should perform a minimum of 20 primary operations a year).

Disadvantages of MCNs and centralization of services

- Patients need to travel further
- Patients of lower income or with poor access to transport are less likely to take up the service
- Training in certain specialities will rely on working within a particular hospital.

NHS initiatives and reforms

There are a number of key NHS reforms and initiatives that although you are not expected to know in great detail, you should be aware of. It is important that before the interview you are abreast of any controversies and it is advisable to flick through publications such as *BMA News*, *BMJ*, *GMC News* and *Hospital Doctor* in the final stages of preparation.

National Service Framework

You should be able to give a definition as well as an example of a national service framework in relation to your speciality.

National service frameworks (NSFs) are long-term strategies for improving specific areas of care. They:

- Set national standards and identify key interventions for a defined service or care group
- Put in place strategies/programmes to support implementation
- Establish ways to ensure progress within an agreed time scale.

The aim of NSFs is to improve standards of care and reduce the variability in service encountered across the NHS, the so-called 'postcode lottery'. Each framework is produced by the Department of Health with the aid of an external reference group (ERG) composed of health professionals, patients, carers, managers and other agencies. NSFs currently exist in the following areas of healthcare:

- Coronary heart disease
- Cancer
- Paediatric intensive care
- Mental health
- Older people
- Diabetes
- Long term conditions
- Renal services

- Children
- Chronic obstructive pulmonary disease (COPD)
- Pharmaceutical industry involvement with NSFs.

Associated question

- What role do NSFs on your clinical practice?

For a useful link, see the Department of Health National Service Frameworks website (www.dh.gov.uk/en/Policyandguidance/Healthandsocialcaretopics/DH_4070951).

NHS targets

National NHS targets are related to NHS national priorities (as determined by the Department of Health) and have been used exhaustively in the NHS as a mechanism to drive continuous improvement in the quality of healthcare delivered.

The Healthcare Commission ('the independent watchdog for healthcare in England') is responsible for assessing whether NHS trusts throughout England meet the government's targets for the NHS, as set out in the Department of Health paper *National Standards, Local Action* (DH 2004b).

You should be able to give an example of a target that you have encountered and be able to discuss the impact on your practice. An obvious example would be the A&E 4-hour. In 2002, prior to the introduction of the 4-hour A&E target, 23% of patients spent in excess of 4 hours within the A&E department; by 2004 this figure fell to 5.3%.

Criticisms of targets

- Results in gaming, e.g., elective operations being cancelled to house 'A&E' patients, holding of patients in ambulances to prevent breaching, etc.
- Demoralizes and places staff under undue pressure
- Skews clinical priorities – i.e., diverts care from patients with greater need
- Leads to micromanagement of the NHS
- Compromises patient care
- Leads to less flexibility – i.e., trusts are less able to respond to local priorities.

Associated questions

- What do you think of hospital league tables?
- What are your views on the publication of individual surgeon or clinician performance data?

The NHS Plan (2000)

The NHS Plan (DH 2000a) is a 10-year process of reform which sets out 'to give the people of Britain a health service fit for the 21st century: a health service designed around the patient'.

Following public consultation, it was established that the public wanted:

- More and better paid staff using new ways of working
- Reduced waiting times
- High quality patient-centred care
- Improvements to local hospitals and surgeries.

Key objectives and areas targeted in *The NHS Plan* (DH 2000a) included:

- The development of national standards, the achievement of which would be monitored by the Commission for Health Improvement (CHI)
- Establishment of the National Institute for Clinical Excellence to ensure cost effectiveness of treatments
- Establishment of an NHS Modernisation Agency to disseminate best practice
- Greater freedom for local NHS organizations that perform well to run their own affairs
- Social services and the NHS to pool resources to prevent patients 'falling between the gap'
- Modern contracts for both GPs and hospital doctors
- Extended roles for nurses and other staff, e.g., the creation of more nurse consultants
- Establishment of a new leadership centre to develop a new generation of managerial and clinical leaders, e.g., 'modern matrons'
- Increased patient representation and rights, e.g., patient advocates within every hospital
- Better use of private sector facilities by the NHS – where this provides value for money and maintains standards of patient care
- Reduced waiting times for treatment through recruitment of extra staff. Examples included:
  - All patients to have a GP appointment within 48 hours, by 2004
  - Reduction of waits in accident and emergency departments
  - A maximum waiting time for outpatient appointments of 3 months and inpatient appointments of 6 months, by 2005
- Greater focus on the treatment of cancer, heart disease and mental health services, e.g., expansion of cancer screening programmes and an end to the postcode lottery in the prescribing of cancer drugs; development of rapid access chest pain clinics nationally by 2003

- Better and new services for the elderly, e.g., nursing care in nursing homes to be free; development of intermediate care services to allow older people to live more independently
- Attempts to address national inequalities through establishments of targets, e.g., to improve the diet of young children by making fruit free in schools for 4–6 year olds.

The NHS Improvement Plan (2004)

The NHS Improvement Plan (DH 2004c) builds upon the commitments of *The NHS Plan* (DH 2000a) and sets out the next stages of the government's NHS modernisation agenda from 2004 to 2008.

The NHS Improvement Plan focuses on:

- Putting patients first by producing more 'responsive, convenient high-quality personalized' patient care
- Health and well-being as a whole, not simply illness
- Further devolution of decision making to local organizations.
  Key initiatives within *The NHS Improvement Plan* include:
- Greater *patient choice*: Right to choose from at least four to five different healthcare providers by 2005 and any provider by 2008
- Greater *support in the community* and at home for managing chronic diseases, e.g., diabetes, heart disease and asthma, with the introduction of:
  ○ Specialist nurses and GPs with special expertise in the condition to reduce emergency hospital admissions
  ○ The Expert Patients Programme – to empower patients to manage their own healthcare.
- Emphasis on *prevention* of disease and tackling inequalities. For example:
  ○ Reduction of death rates for the under 75s from heart diseases and stroke by at least 40% by 2010
  ○ Reduction of death rates from cancer and suicides by 20% (from 1997) to 2010.
- *Reduction in waiting time* – 18 weeks from referral to treatment
- *Greater involvement of the independent sector* – to provide up to 15% of procedures on behalf of the NHS to support capacity and choice
- *PCTs to commission care from a wider range of providers*, including independent sector organizations, e.g., independent sector treatment centres (ISTCs) and NHS treatment centres (i.e., practice-based commissioning).
- *Information systems*
  ○ Enabling patients to choose care at their convenience by 2005 – i.e., 'Choose and Book'
  ○ Electronic prescriptions

  ○ NHS Direct, NHS Direct Online and NHS Digital Television
  ○ Electronic health records.
- *Financial incentives and performance management* to drive delivery of *The NHS Improvement Plan*:
  ○ Payment by results
  ○ Primary care trusts to develop incentives for GPs to deliver higher quality care
  ○ Money, control and responsibility to be handed over to local health services, e.g., practice-based commissioning and NHS foundation trusts
  ○ Primary care trusts to control over 80% of the NHS budget.

ISTCs: independent sector involvement in the NHS

Independent sector treatment centres (ISTCs) are privately funded units commissioned by PCTs (which can tender in competition with NHS trusts for contracts) to provide specific services for NHS patients. They are often situated in the same geographical locality as the hospital and tend to carry out procedures that are relatively simple, straightforward and which should have few complications, e.g., inguinal hernia repairs, endoscopy, cataract surgery. At the outset the medical staff were brought in from the continent to avoid poaching staff from the NHS and to enable ISTCs to set their own financial tariff; however, more recently, it has been agreed that NHS consultants can contract to work sessionally within their local ISTC.

The theory behind ISTCs is that they could perform minor and intermediary operations with a higher turnover in comparison to NHS trusts as – unlike in the NHS – the number of elective beds would be guaranteed, due to the absence of emergency or long-stay patients, leading to both improved patient access to care and a reduction in waiting times. *The NHS Improvement Plan* aims to have 15% of NHS-funded operations carried out by the independent sector by 2008.

Disadvantages of ISTCs

- They cherry-pick straightforward cases, leaving more complicated operations for NHS trusts to manage (i.e. they have an atypical case mix)
- They take away training and teaching opportunities; do not follow up patients
- NHS trust are left to manage any complications that arise (not the operating surgeon); in addition, no follow-up of patients is offered
- Preferential contracts have previously been offered to ISTCs, which have put NHS trusts at a disadvantage

- There is a loss of income from the NHS to the private sector, since the money from PCTs follow the patient (PBR)
- They lack formal mechanisms regarding clinical governance
- They have higher complication rates compared to NHS treatment centres (HPERU 2005).

In preparation for the interviews you should find out more about a local ISTC.

Foundation hospitals

NHS foundation trusts (also known as 'foundation hospitals') form part of the government's NHS reforms outlined in *The NHS Plan* (DH 2000a), and are independent, public benefit corporations which, although part of the NHS, have a greater freedom and flexibility in managing their affairs compared to non-foundation NHS trusts.

NHS trusts that score the maximum three stars in the annual star ratings for hospital performance have been invited to apply for foundation status. Gaining foundation status allows trusts to tailor care and be more responsive to the needs of the local population, since:

- Decision making is devolved from central government control to local organizations and communities, giving greater power to local communities and front-line staff
- They are accountable to local communities, not central government
- They have financial freedoms to borrow money or raise capital through private finance initiatives (PFIs)
- They have freedom to invest in developing new local services and innovations
- They are able to establish stronger connections with those living in the community as the members of the trust's Board of Governors are drawn from patients, public and staff
- They support patient choice by increasing the diversity and number of service providers.

NHS foundation trusts remain firmly part of the NHS and are subject to NHS standards, performance ratings and systems of inspection.

Criticisms of foundation trusts

- Goes against the spirit of the NHS
- Is back-door privatization of the NHS
- Leads to a two-tier system, increasing health inequalities
- Leads to no real improvement in quality of care delivered (Lewis & Hinton 2005).

Connecting for Health and the NHS National Programme for Information Technology (NPfIT)

Connecting for Health was established in April 2005 as the single national IT provider for the NHS, with the primary role of delivering the National Programme for IT (NPfIT) by 2014.

The National Programme for IT (DH 2002b) aims to improve patient care by enabling clinicians and other NHS staff to increase their efficiency and effectiveness through improved access to patient information via new computer systems and services.

The key initiatives are:

- *The NHS Care Records Service (NHS CRS)*: Delivery of a centralized electronic database of patient medical records for all NHS patients which are available and can be accessed by NHS staff wherever a patient is being treated in the UK
- *Choose and Book* (see below)
- *Electronic Transfer of Prescriptions (ETP), through the Electronic Prescription Service (EPS)*: The paper-based system will be replaced with an electronic version, which will allow patients to pick up repeat prescriptions from any pharmacy in the country via fast computer network links between NHS organizations
- *Picture Archiving and Communications Systems (PACS)*: These systems – which enable digital images such as scans and x-rays to be stored and accessed electronically – have already been successfully introduced, and are now available not only within hospital trusts but also to GPs who are networked to the local system and to some clinicians at home, e.g., radiologists
- *NHSmail*: An NHS email and directory service – i.e., the NHS 'intranet'.

Criticisms of Connecting for Health

- Failed to engage and involve frontline staff in its development
- Long delays in its implementation – unrealistic timetable
- Expensive with spiralling costs (total bill may be in excess of £20 billion)
- Concerns regarding security of data and patient confidentiality.

Associated question

- What are the advantages and disadvantages of computerized health records?

Choose and Book

'Choose and Book' (also known as CaB or C&B) is a national, secure, electronically based referral service, which allows patients to book their first outpatient appointment with a specialist, at a hospital of their choice, at the time and date of their choosing. Choose and Book was initially introduced in 2005 in the NHS National Programme for IT (NPfIT). Appointments can be booked through the patient's GP or by the patient at home by telephone or over the internet, following the agreement by the GP of the appropriateness of the referral.

Choose and Book is to be harnessed as a tool to both measure and deliver the government's 18-week target from referral to treatment of non-urgent conditions.

Advantages

- Greater patient choice (can choose up to four hospitals)
- Convenient (patients can choose when – i.e., schedule appointments around other appointments)
- Ability to cancel or change appointments electronically, thus potentially reduces DNA (Did Not Attend) rates
- Engages patients in the decision-making process
- Reduces delays as patients can select hospitals with shorter waiting lists
- Allows tracking of referrals – referrals can no longer be 'lost in the system'.

Disadvantages

- Additional workload for clinicians
- Open to inappropriate use
- Potentially liable to breaches in security.

For useful website links, see www.chooseandbook.nhs.uk (Choose and Book) and www.nhschoicespreview.nhs.uk (NHS Choices).

Strategic Health Authorities

There are 10 Strategic Health Authorities (SHAs) across England. SHAs are charged with the responsibility of managing the NHS locally, providing strategic leadership and facilitating development and improvement. In addition, SHAs provide a key link between the Department of Health and the NHS, and are responsible for holding local NHS organizations, e.g., NHS trusts, accountable for delivery of key government reform policies, e.g., *The NHS Improvement Plan.*

Primary Care Trusts

There have been a huge number of changes in the funding arrangements within the NHS over the last few years.

Primary Care Trust (PCT) is the collective term used to describe a group of GP practices. A PCT is defined as: 'a legal entity, set up by order of the Secretary of State. It is a free-standing NHS body, performance managed by a Strategic Health Authority (SHA). The overall function of a Primary Care Trust is to improve the health of the community; develop primary and community health services; and commission secondary care services.' (NHS Information Authority 2003).

There are 152 PCTs in England and they are able to negotiate and commission services from NHS hospitals and the private sector under a national service contract. PCTs are responsible for 80% of NHS spending, which is equivalent to around £58 billion.

Practice-Based Commissioning

Management questions, such as those related to practice-based commissioning, require an understanding and appreciation of the financial flows within the NHS.

Practice-based commissioning (PBC) was introduced in 2005, and forms a key part of the government's NHS reform policy. It is intended to give more decision-making power over NHS resources to general practitioners with the prime objective of delivering more cost-effective and convenient forms of treatment *outside* hospitals.

Prior to the introduction of PBC, the majority of NHS funding flowed from the Department of Health to primary care trusts (PCTs) who subsequently paid hospitals, GPs and other healthcare providers for the services delivered locally. Under PBC, GPs are set a budget by their PCT and given detailed financial and clinical activity data regarding how they manage their patients, including comparisons with other practices locally and nationally. This data is intended to guide GPs to commission new services or use existing providers to provide cost-effective care. The incentive for GP practices is that they are allowed to keep a proportion of any 'efficiency gains'. Increased cost-effective PBC is central to delivering a number of other key objectives:

- Greater patient choice due to a greater diversity of providers
- More convenient 'care closer to home' – i.e., not within hospitals (DH 2006b)
- Achievement of the 18-week 'referral to treatment' waiting time target (DH 2006b) through service redesign, e.g., new diagnostic equipment within the community

- Better preventive care due to greater freedom and incentives for GPs to look after patients within the practice-setting – thus emergency hospital admissions for chronic diseases such as asthma and diabetes may be avoided
- Reduction in the number of GP referrals to secondary care (hospitals), e.g., through the establishment of referral management centres and the encouragement of GPs to develop specialist interests
- Reducing inequalities to accessing care.

(See also other important areas within this section, in Further reading.)

Payment by Results

Payment by results (PBR) is a system of reimbursement introduced in 2003 in an attempt to increase efficiency and transparency in the hospital sector. In this system, each condition treated has a specific nationally defined coding that will determine the amount of money the hospital will receive – i.e., a fixed tariff for each completed episode (e.g., each outpatient appointment, investigation and treatment procedure).

The funding or 'payment' comes from either the general practice or the PCT and thus money within the NHS follows the patient and hospitals with high quality activity are rewarded. A key criticism of PBR, however, is that the vast majority of these episodes are undertariffed, which results in hospitals participating in the scheme losing out financially. In addition, it has the potential to financially destabilize NHS Trusts.

You do not need to know a great detail about PBR; however, if this is an area that you are interested in, you would be well advised to talk to one of the accountants within your trust.

Referral Management Schemes

Referral Management Schemes (RMS) – such as Clinical Assessment Services (CAS), Clinical Assessment and Treatment Services (CATS) and Integrated Clinical Assessment and Treatment Services (ICATS) – were introduced following the government's White Paper *Our Health, Our Care, Our Say* (DH 2006b), and is a term which describes 'all arrangements that incorporate any intermediary level(s) of triage, assessment and treatment between traditional primary and secondary care including paper-based screening systems (or their electronic equivalent)'. Their aim is to 'improve the patient-care pathway to deliver tangible benefits for patients' (BMA 2007).

Advantages

- Reduces waiting times for non-urgent cases (waiting times for urgent cases are not affected)
- Cost effective
- Tracks referral patterns.

Disadvantages

- May be used by PCTs as a method for rationing services (both first and follow-up appointments) into secondary care
- Waiting times may be prolonged due to the financial constraints i.e., if the PCT does not have the money to fund a particular service, it may not be made available
- Could limit patient choice
- Leads to a loss of clinical autonomy – as there is a managerial rather than a clinical basis for referrals
- May compromise patient confidentiality.

Improving Working Lives

Improving Working Lives (IWL) is a Department of Health initiative which aims to encourage employers to develop a range of human resources (HR), policies and practices which supports staff, promotes their welfare and development, and helps them to achieve a healthy work–life balance.

The IWL standard (DH 2000b) is a model of good HR practice against which NHS employers are assessed. If the IWL standard is achieved, the organization is accredited with an IWL kite mark.

Examples of performance measures used to assess an employer's commitment to IWL include:

- Development of HR strategy to support service targets
- Commitment to: childcare support; reduced hours options; flexitime; career breaks; flexible retirement
- Building of a diverse workforce that reflects the local community; evidence of commitment to a healthy workplace
- Accessibility to training and development packages.

NHS Direct

NHS Direct is the national telephone healthcare advice service operated by nurses using decision support software to provide consistent clinical criteria and was launched in 1998. Its aim is to provide information and advice about health, illness and health services to enable patients to make decisions about their healthcare and that of their families (NHS Direct Mission Statement).

Key notes on NHS Direct

- Consists of a website, 24-hour telephone line and interactive digital television service
- >2 million people access NHS Direct each month.

Advantages

- Safe – 29 adverse event cases in 3 years (National Audit Office 2002)
- Encourages more appropriate use of healthcare services, e.g., GPs, A&E
- Has a high caller satisfaction.

Disadvantages

- Can be delays of up to 30 minutes to answer calls
- Not accessed equally by all social groups – poorer uptake amongst elderly (>65 years), ethnic minorities, disabled and low socioeconomic groups.

Agenda for Change

Agenda for Change (DH 2004d) aims to create a fairer pay scheme, increasing harmony within the NHS and leading to greater links between career and pay progression. Following assessment under the NHS Job Evaluation Scheme, staff are placed on one of nine pay bands. *Agenda for Change* was implemented in the NHS for all NHS staff, except doctors, dentists and some senior managers, in 2004.

Further questions

- What would you do if you were Health Minister for 1 day?
- How would convince your trust that a procedure you would like to introduce is cost effective?
- What are PFIs?
- What are your views on the Darzi Report (*Healthcare for London: A Framework for Action*)?

Clinical experience, motivation and personality

The aim of this part of the interview is to ascertain your suitability in terms of competencies achieved for entry into specialist training.

The interview panel will essentially be looking for specific qualities as stated in the person specification for the post, namely:

- Clinical knowledge and expertise
  - Appropriate knowledge base
  - Capacity to apply sound clinical judgement to problems
  - Ability to prioritize clinical need
  - Awareness of the basics of managing acutely ill patients
- Vigilance and situational awareness
  - Capacity to be alert to dangers or problems
  - Capacity to monitor developing situations and anticipate issues
- Coping with pressure
  - Capacity to operate under pressure
  - Initiative and resilience to cope with setbacks and adapt to rapidly changing circumstances
  - Awareness of own limitations and knows when to ask for help
- Managing others and team involvement
  - Capacity to work cooperatively with others
  - Ability to work effectively in multi-professional teams
  - Leadership skills
- Problem solving and decision making
  - Capacity to solve problems
  - Ability to make decisions
- Empathy and sensitivity
  - Capacity to take in others' perspectives and treat others with understanding
  - Sees patients as people
- Communication skills
  - Demonstrates clarity in written/spoken communication
  - Adapts language as appropriate to the situation
  - Able to build rapport, listen, persuade and negotiate
- Organization and planning
  - Capacity to organize oneself, prioritize own work and organize ward rounds
  - Demonstrates punctuality, preparation and self-discipline
  - Possesses basic IT skills
- Professional integrity and respect for others
  - Capacity to take responsibility for own actions
  - Demonstrates a non-judgemental approach towards others
  - Displays honesty, integrity, awareness of confidentiality and ethical issues
  - Possesses delegation skills

- Learning and personal development
  - Demonstrates interest and realistic insight into speciality
  - Demonstrates self-awareness
  - Ability to accept feedback
  - Extracurricular activities/achievements relevant to acute medicine.

Clinical knowledge and expertise

The interviewers will expect to have a copy of your CV which you should provide from your portfolio and they will, of course, have your application form. The first panel member is likely to ask you to discuss the clinical experience that you have gained to date, and the question is likely to be phrased: 'Tell me about your clinical experience to date.' or 'Tell us about your postgraduate training.' For the more experienced candidate applying at a higher level, you may be asked for your experience in a confined time limit, e.g., 'Tell us about your clinical experience during the last 2 years.'

Remember that the interviewer does not want to hear a list of hospitals and dates of when you worked there. They want you to take them through your personal story. If it is complex, for example if you have clearly changed speciality during your training, or you have taken time-out, you need to be able to explain the reasons for this. Alternatively, the interviewers may decide to pick one or two jobs out and ask you about these in more detail. It is usual with these types of questions for the interviewer to allow you to just keep talking and the advice would be that if no one interrupts you, you should do just that. As long as you are talking sense and not making statements that are factually wrong or omitting key facts, then from your point of view, the fewer the interruptions, the fewer questions that you will be asked and the higher the score that you should obtain. You need, however, to practise answering this type of question.

Importantly, at a junior level, it is more appropriate in your answer to refer to the consultants you have worked for by their title, e.g., Professor John Smith, Mr John Smith, Mr William Appleyard, Dr Ken Brown, etc. Familiarity by calling the consultant in the interview John Smith or simply John etc. may not portray you in the best light.

Talking about your posts

It is best practice to discuss all the positive things that you have gained out of each of your posts. Remember, however, that the interview process is also probing into your approach to training and if a particular post was weak in one area, e.g., endoscopy, then it is perfectly reasonable for you to express and acknowledge this to the panel, but it would be much better if you could use that as a justification to move onto the next job which may have actually been stronger in that particular area, e.g., 'My exposure to [x] was poor in this post. However, in my next job there was more than ample opportunity to remedy this deficiency in my training.' This makes it appear that you are planning your career sensibly. Of course, the panel members all realize that many trainees will have gone through a set rotation; however, acknowledging the strengths and weaknesses of each individual job, whilst showing how they balance out throughout the rotation, is often a good way of discussing the merits of each individual post as well as your overall clinical experience obtained.

'What procedures/operations would you feel competent in performing when on-call?'

Your response to this question should reflect the procedures you have performed or assisted in as evidenced by your logbook, which you will be asked to produce at interview.

In addition to assessing your competency/ability to work with or without direct supervision, this question importantly gauges your awareness of your own limitations – i.e., whether you can operate semi-independently whilst being safe. Even if you are not hugely clinically experienced, this can be largely circumvented by enthusiasm and a clear motivation to learn.

In this part of the interview it is likely that your logbook will be reviewed and you may be asked to describe procedures that you have performed yourself, as well those in which you have assisted.

Approaching clinical scenarios

The second half of this section of the interview will often be related to clinical scenarios. There are obviously a huge number of clinical scenarios which can be used and the choice of scenario will depend on your clinical experience and the speciality you are applying to. Most scenarios will however be based upon real incidents.

The general approach is to listen carefully to the clinical scenario. The age of the patient may be very important. The symptoms and signs will undoubtedly be important, as will any underlying medical disorders.

There appear to be two different approaches taken to clinical scenarios by candidates:

- One group of candidates will spend the first few minutes asking about or requesting additional information relating to the patient, e.g., age, co-morbidity, etc. This is often unnecessary and can sometimes result in a rather irritating dialogue that goes on for several minutes whilst additional symptoms or signs that the trainee would like are given.

- The second approach is to discuss the clinical scenario as it has been given. But, of course, if, for instance, no age has been given, then say during the discussion that there may be variations according to the age of the patient, and that if the patient is over 65 the approach may be somewhat different from that if the patient is aged 30, and then discuss the approach for each age group. This keeps you, as the interviewee, in charge and talking and, again, results in fewer interruptions. Thus – provided that you are talking sense – should mean that you will achieve a high score.

If you forget something, you should acknowledge this. It will usually be quite apparent to the panel members that this is just a short memory lapse and when they prompt you, you can get back into full swing. Do not leave large time gaps with silence while you try to think of something. It is much better to say that you have forgotten or that you do not know, and to move on to the next topic, rather than to just sit there in silence.

Remember with the clinical scenarios that there is often more than one way to deal with the case but the fundamentals remain the same.

Management means taking a history, examining the patient, formulating a differential diagnosis, investigating the patient, formulating a definitive diagnosis and treating the patient. If you are asked how to treat a patient with a given diagnosis, then you may assume that that diagnosis is correct and you should deal merely with the treatment.

However, as we all know, sometimes people say treatment when they really mean management. If you are asked how you would treat a patient, and the diagnosis is not clear, it would be best to say, 'Having gone through the history and examination and formulated a differential diagnosis of … [give a list of the possible differential diagnoses] … and having then investigated the patient and established a definitive diagnosis of … [give the diagnosis], I would proceed to treat the patient.' This will allow the interviewer to interrupt and say, 'Oh no, tell me a little bit more about the history etc,' if he has inadvertently said treatment but really means management. The same is true if someone asks you how you manage a particular disease process. You should always start with history, examination, etc. If the interviewer wishes you to go straight to treatment he will interrupt and say, 'No, no, no, let's proceed straight to treatment', and that way time is not wasted.

Common clinical scenarios

These will depend upon the speciality to which you are applying. In the weeks before interview you should prepare yourself by going through clinical cases that you have seen or ones that you believe may be important as the scenarios will be based upon real cases. In general terms, they will either deal with acute or chronic conditions and the wording of the scenario will often give you clues as to what the interviewer is trying to probe from you.

Example: Tell me about how you would manage an 85-year-old diabetic with a 5-day history of vomiting and abdominal pain.

Here you can see that the discussion will relate to the resuscitation of an elderly person whose fluid requirements will need to be carefully monitored. The diabetes will also need to be managed and this is an important part of the scenario. In addition, the 5 days of vomiting will lead to a number of metabolic changes and this will dictate the type of resuscitation.

In patients requiring fluid resuscitation, often the interviewer is trying to establish your understanding of fluid management including when (i.e., under what circumstances) and how you would monitor fluid balance, e.g., the use of a central venous pressure (CVP) line. It is often the use of CVP monitoring that is poorly discussed by trainees, even though they probably have a good understanding and experience of this area.

Finally, the statement 'abdominal pain' indicates that you should following the initial management, discuss establishment of the diagnosis and treatment.

Other clinical scenarios may relate to more generic, practical procedures, such as insertion of a central venous pressure catheter, or even male catheterization.

Medical and surgical emergencies

- 'A patient presents with peritonitis post colonoscopy. How would you manage them?' (Sigmoid perforation post colonoscopy requiring laparotomy and sigmoid colectomy)
- 'How would you manage a patient presenting with acute onset lower limb weakness, lower limb sensory disturbance and urinary retention?' (Spinal cord compression or cauda equina syndrome requiring urgent MRI and referral to the neurosurgeons)
- 'How would you manage a patient presenting with a severe headache, fever, nausea ± vomiting, photophobia, neck stiffness?' (Meningitis)
- 'You are asked to review a patient who is hypotensive and has a haemoglobin of 4.7 g/dl post laparoscopic cholecystectomy. How would you tackle the situation?' (Postoperative bleeding requiring resuscitation and urgent surgical exploration)

The above scenarios are all examples of medical or surgical emergencies which require early recognition and intervention. You should state this in your opening sentence. Each scenario requires you to identify the most likely or important differential diagnosis (given in parentheses for the above examples) and you should demonstrate a logical approach and understanding of the management of each particular condition in your answer.

The interviewer essentially is trying to establish whether you are safe and whether you have had hands-on experience or the skills necessary to cope with the level of entry into specialist training to which you are applying. In essence, will you be a coherent, sensible voice at the end of the phone at 2 o'clock in the morning?

In general, your management of the patient should include resuscitation, history, examination and the appropriate investigations, which will guide your further treatment. Importantly, you should demonstrate a multi-disciplinary approach to the patient's care, involving other specialists (e.g., radiologists, neurosurgeons, anaesthetists) and your seniors/consultant as appropriate. You should not be afraid to ask for help.

Try to answer each scenario as if you were actually there. For example: 'How do you manage a patient in A&E with an acutely ischaemic leg?'

- 'This is a surgical emergency. I would resuscitate the patient and my further management would include taking a full history, examining the patient and performing the appropriate investigations.'
- 'Acute limb ischaemia can be caused by a thrombus or an embolus and this would affect my management of the patient. In the history I would want to determine the onset of symptoms (6-hour rule) and associated symptoms such as pain, pallor, perishing coldness, paraesthesia and paralysis. A history of intermittent claudication, rest pain and significant risk factors for peripheral vascular disease … would suggest acute on chronic disease and perhaps a thrombus … On examination …' etc.

The discussion is likely to continue onto the investigations, and in the surgical specialities it would not be unreasonable to discuss the intervention/operation itself.

Importantly, when asked to discuss the operation you should talk about:

- Obtaining patient consent
- Marking the appropriate side preoperatively
- The type of anaesthetic
- Positioning the patient
- Shaving the operative area if relevant
- Scrubbing and prepping the patient
- The technical aspects of the procedure
- Postoperative care, e.g., HDU, ITU, iv heparin, etc.

Questions requiring prioritization of patients

Example: You have two patients in A&E admitted at the same time. One with a suspected ruptured abdominal aortic aneurysm, a second with peritonitis and your FY1 is concerned about an unwell patient on the ward. How would you tackle the situation?

This type of multi-faceted question is useful for selecting out the more capable candidates. The aim of this type of question is several-fold and it can serve to assess your ability to:

- Communicate
- Act under pressure
- Rapidly assess and prioritize patients, and recognize sick patients who require your immediate attention
- Work as a team
- Act as a team leader and coordinate the efforts of other members of the team
- Recognize your limits and to ask for help from other specialist teams, e.g., anaesthetists, intensivists, surgeons, medics on-call and your seniors – this includes your consultant.

It is important to recognize with this type of question that you cannot be in more than one place at the same time and nor are you expected to be. However, using effective communication and calling for help early, as well as delegating tasks (e.g., ask your FY1 where appropriate to involve the medics or HDU/ITU), the scenario may be managed successfully with no detrimental impact on patient care.

Other common clinically orientated questions

'How would you obtain informed consent for a procedure?'

Consent is often an important part of clinical scenarios and is of particular importance to those specialities where invasive procedures or interventions are commonplace.

There are many questions that can be asked in relation to consent and often they will relate to a particular procedure and often one that you will be familiar with as evidenced by your logbook. Questions on consent are one way of discussing how well the trainee understands the intervention, including the benefits of the intervention as well as its associated complications.

Principles of obtaining consent

When describing complications during consent you should discuss the common complications and, importantly, all those with an incidence of greater than 1%. *Consent should only be taken from the patient by a person capable of performing that procedure independently.* However, all trainees should be aware of the principles of obtaining informed consent:

- Informed consent can only be obtained from patients who have the mental capacity to give consent and patients under the age of 16 years need a parent's informed consent.
- Informed consent may be either verbal or written and relies on the patient being given a full explanation of the procedure/investigation (including any prior work-up and their management post procedure) and its expected benefits and risks. The patient should be able to understand the procedure and be able to reason. It is therefore important to avoid medical jargon, to ensure that the patient has understood what they have been told and to give the patient sufficient time to both ask questions and finally reach a decision.
- Where alternative options are available the patient should be made aware of these.
- In some instances an interpreter may be required.

Importantly, in the absence of the patient's consent to treatment, a doctor (even if well-intentioned) can be sued for or charged with battery or assault.

It is useful before the interview to obtain a copy of the consent form as used in your own hospital and to read through it very carefully and understand each section. All consent forms are in general the same but there are slight differences, e.g., not all include consent for tissues to be used for research purposes. (See also the Clinical knowledge and expertise section in Further reading.)

Difficult questions on consent

The question may be made more difficult by changing the course of the discussion to include obtaining consent from patients who are vulnerable, e.g., some elderly patients, psychiatric patients, young patients, patients who are temporarily not in a position to understand the procedure fully e.g., due to sepsis.

Children and consent

There is no defined age at which a child is regarded as competent to consent and those 16 years and older should be regarded as competent unless proven otherwise. Importantly, any competent young person, regardless of age, can independently seek medical advice and give valid consent to medical treatment. Parental consent is not necessary and the young person's ability to understand is the factor that renders them competent. However, where possible it is always better to have parental support.

Gillick competence and the Fraser ruling

Gillick competence is a standard originating from English medical law and is used to determine whether a child (16 years or younger) is able to consent to his or her own medical treatment, without the permission or knowledge of their parents.

Gillick competence arose as a concept following the case of *Gillick v West Norfolk and Wisbech Area Health Authority* (1985) in which Mrs Victoria Gillick challenged the Department of Health guidance which advised that a doctor could give girls under the age of 16 years contraceptive advice and treatment without the consent, involvement or knowledge of their parents. The judge ruled against Mrs Gillick, stating that, 'As a matter of Law the parental right to determine whether or not their minor child below the age of sixteen will have medical treatment terminates if and when the child achieves sufficient understanding and intelligence to understand fully what is proposed.'

The question of the rights of children under 16 years of age to consent to treatment on their own behalf was reviewed by Lord Fraser in 1985 in connection with contraception and has become known as the 'Fraser ruling'. As a result the law does not specify an age below which a health professional cannot give treatment or contraceptive advice provided the health professional feels that the young person can understand the advice given. A young person under 16 years of age who is thought to be competent to give consent should be referred to as 'Fraser-ruling competent'. Previously we would have used the term 'Gillick-competent'.

Difficult questions on consent regarding children

In the case of abortion the Medical Defence Union advises that if a request for abortion is made by a girl under 16, her parents should be consulted unless the girl forbids the health professional to do so. Best practice would be to obtain the patient's consent and the written authority of the parents; however, parental refusal would not allow a perfectly lawful abortion to go ahead if the patient herself consents provided the health professional is clear that the patient is mature enough to understand the nature of the operation and competent to give consent.

Where parental refusal to treatment has occurred it would be unlawful for a health professional to proceed with treatment if the child is not considered Fraser-ruling competent. Occasionally parental wishes conflict with reasonable medical practice and if it is deemed that this is not in the best interests of the child then advice would be to obtain a second opinion and possibly seek application to the court.

Life-saving procedures on a child in the face of parental refusal are unlikely to be questioned although it is important that the child's best interests must always be uppermost. A difficult example would be the case of blood transfusion in a child with Jehovah's Witness parents. Here again a second opinion would be favoured as well as early application to the court. If, during the interview, you are unsure of the exact legal position, in any given scenario, then you should say so. It is always better to admit that you do not know something rather than try to make it up in such difficult circumstances.

'What do you understand by the term "Duty of Care"?'

The 'Duties of a Doctor' are outlined in the GMC's guidance *Good Medical Practice* (GMC 2006b) and states that as a doctor you must:

- Make the care of your patient your first concern
- Protect and promote the health of patients and the public
- Provide a good standard of practice and care
  - Keep your professional knowledge and skills up to date
  - Recognize and work within the limits of your competence
  - Work with colleagues in the ways that best serve patients' interests
- Treat patients as individuals and respect their dignity
  - Treat patients politely and considerately
  - Respect patients' right to confidentiality
- Work in partnership with patients
  - Listen to patients and respond to their concerns and preferences
  - Give patients the information they want or need in a way they can understand
  - Respect patients' right to reach decisions with you about their treatment and care
  - Support patients in caring for themselves to improve and maintain their health
- Be honest and open and act with integrity

○ Act without delay if you have good reason to believe that you or a colleague may be putting patients at risk

○ Never discriminate unfairly against patients or colleagues

○ Never abuse your patients' trust in you or the public's trust in the profession.

Importantly, 'You are personally accountable for your professional practice and must always be prepared to justify your decisions and actions.'

'What is the difference between a guideline and a protocol?'

A protocol is a strict set of rules or procedures; a guideline is desired good or best practice. Acceptance of the latter is voluntary. In clinical practice, guidelines are developed to help or assist healthcare professionals and patients to make decisions; this may relate to prevention, treatment or screening.

'What is an integrated care pathway?'

Integrated care pathways (ICPs) are structured, multi-disciplinary care plans which detail the essential steps in the care of a patient with a specific clinical problem. ICPs are commonplace within the NHS and exist for >45 conditions in a number of specialities, e.g., acute stroke, orthopaedics and rehabilitation medicine, palliative care (e.g., Care of the Dying pathways), mental health, paediatrics and general surgery.

The perceived benefits of ICPs are that they:

● Are patient focused
● Standardize patient care
● Support the implementation of national guidelines
● Reduce the length of hospital stay
● Improve patient data collection
● Improve communication as they involve a multi-disciplinary approach
● Reduce complaints as patients are better informed as to what to expect during their stay in hospital and following discharge
● Reduce the need for follow-up in clinics
● Reduce cost – as both length of stay and need for follow-up are reduced.

The disadvantages of ICPs are that they can be time-consuming to develop and implement and they require the cooperation of all members of the multi-disciplinary team.

Other questions

- What attributes do you have that make you suitable for entry at ST1/ST2/ST3?
- Describe your most interesting case to date and what you learnt from it.
- Summarize the evidence of your clinical skills and expertise in relation to this speciality. What have you found most challenging and why? What areas do you need to improve?
- How would you triage someone out in the field?

Behavioural questions

Assessment of the qualities in the person specification may be assessed using situational or behavioural questions in addition to, or as part of, more generic questions.

Work-related behavioural or situational questions are becoming increasingly more popular in medicine and are used to assess your performance in the past, the theory being that past performance is often the best predictor of future performance in a similar situation. Situational questions are thought to be more objective than traditional questions and following an often very open-ended starting question; the interviewer will then probe deeper with further questions, e.g., 'How did you feel at the time?'

In terms of preparation, you should practise your story-telling abilities and although the number of potential situational questions that could arise is exhaustive, it is useful to think of a handful of scenarios beforehand which can be adapted to cover the most common questions or which demonstrate the necessary key person specification qualities. Each story (answer) should be specific and incorporate some background/scene-setting information (this should be brief), the specific action you took (which demonstrates a specific quality within the person specification) and the positive outcome. An example of a situational question would be, 'Describe a time when you have had to coordinate the activities of a team in a critical situation and how you dealt with the stress.' You should use 'real' examples in your responses, and avoid embellishing the truth or exaggerating, as any experienced interviewer will easily spot this.

Generic questions

There are a lot of questions that crop up during the interview which may be used either as an opening question or may follow from something mentioned. A number of these so-called generic questions are discussed below in the context of the desired or essential qualities within the person specification.

Vigilance and situational awareness

Common questions

- Describe an example from your experience in this speciality when applying your clinical judgement had a defining impact on patient management. What did you do and how do you think the outcome was affected by your judgement?

Coping with pressure

Medicine, due to a multitude of factors, e.g., pace, lack of resources, targets, workload, etc., can be incredibly stressful and throughout your career you are likely to have periods where you feel under considerable pressure, and personal circumstances can exacerbate matters. Although a degree of stress and pressure at work can have its advantages (e.g., teaches you to become more organized and prioritize, improves productivity, provides challenges), more importantly, it can have a significant negative impact on your health, emotions and behaviour.

There are a number of different strategies that can be adopted to deal with stress at work and these are likely to be dependent on both your personality and the specific situation.

Common questions in this area usually expect you to demonstrate your ability to cope under pressure and discuss the mechanisms you have adopted to do this, e.g., 'How do you deal with stress/pressure?' or 'Can you think of a situation where you were under pressure and how you coped with it?' In the latter you should give an example and reflect on the situation, discussing the strategies you used to successfully or unsuccessfully manage the situation as well as how you may deal with the same/similar situation differently in the future.

General Approach to Tackling Pressure/stress

- Review your current strategies with coping or dealing with stress
- Identify and be aware of the factors that cause you stress
- Recognize stressful factors or situations early
- Identify your goals or tasks which need to be completed
- Be realistic about your deadlines or resources needed
- Select strategies and develop/adapt and maintain a system that works for you
- Obtain feedback from others regarding your progress
- Recognize and reward your achievements
- Lifestyle modifications: factor in regular breaks, sleep, exercise and relaxation time

---

Managing others and team involvement

Common questions

'How do ensure good teamwork?'

The factors that are required for good team working are outlined in the GMC's document *Good Medical Practice* (2006b). In general, good team working relies on ensuring that:

- The skills and contributions of each member of the team are respected
- You listen to and take on board each team member's views
- Communication is effective both within as well as outside the team
- Each member of the team understands their own role as well the role of every other member of the team
- The team's performance is regularly reviewed and any areas for improvement are identified and addressed
- Support is given to team members who are in need/distress.

'What is a team and why is teamwork important?'

A team is a distinguishable set of two or more individuals with complementary skills who interact dynamically and interdependently to achieve a specified shared common performance goal.

Advantages of teamwork

- Improves efficiency and quality of care delivered due to a combined knowledge and skill mix
- Improves staff morale and job satisfaction
- Reduces stress
- Fosters a feeling of ownership in the objective/product
- Provides a supportive environment and encourages learning and personal development
- Improves communication
- Improves quality of decision-making
- Encourages creativity.

'Give an example where you showed leadership.'

Questions about leadership are common. In this question, you will need to describe skills that make a good leader and relate this to specific examples/ situations which demonstrate that you have these skills.

For example:

- A leader leads by example and needs to be enthusiastic, competent and confident …
- A good leader gets respect by setting a good and high standard …
- A good leader understands and motivates his team and understands the strengths and weaknesses of each team member …
- A good leader has clear objectives and aspirations and communicates them to the team …
- A good leader is also flexible …
- A good leader is a decision-maker and can see the reasons for change and will implement these …

Although at a junior level you are not expected to have developed as many of the skills related to good leadership as your more senior colleagues, applicants should be able to demonstrate a clear understanding of the attributes that make a good leader and be seen to be starting to be developing these skills.

You should plan your answer to this question with appropriate examples. Remember also that a good leader praises and encourages other members of their team. Team playing is a very good attribute and much of the questioning around leadership will relate to team players.

Associated questions

- Describe a time where you demonstrated teamwork
- Why are multi-disciplinary teams (MDTs) important? What are the advantages and disadvantages of MDTs?
- Describe a time where you demonstrated leadership
- What makes a good leader?
- The bed manager wants to put a medical patient on a surgical ward and the ward sister is not happy. How would you handle the situation?
- What approach did you take to get the best out of the team? How has this experience developed your ability to direct others effectively?
- What management skills do you possess? (Try to think of examples from both inside and outside medicine.)

Problem-solving and decision-making

Common questions

'How do you deal with a patient who presents with a condition that you are unfamiliar with?'

Your answer should demonstrate that you have the ability to openly admit to patients and colleagues alike that you are unfamiliar with the management of the condition. However, you should have an enthusiastic, clear and resourceful approach to managing the patient, which could include the use of textbooks, the internet and discussion with more senior colleagues or specialist centres. In general, you should utilize all of the resources available to you to try to find out about the condition and how you should manage it.

'Describe an incident when you found it difficult to make an effective judgement in a challenging situation. How did you overcome this difficulty and how has this experience informed your subsequent practice?'

This question is looking for evidence of reflective practice and the answer to this question will be individual to you and depend on your own personal experiences. Possible examples may include:

- Ethical dilemmas, e.g., do not attempt resuscitation (DNAR) orders
- Near misses
- Critical incidence reporting, e.g., drug prescribing errors.

(See also the Problem solving and decision-making section in Further reading.)

Empathy and sensitivity + communication skills

The GMC's document *Good Medical Practice* (2006b) gives guidelines regarding effectively communicating with patients, stating you should:

- Listen to patients
- Ask for and respect their views
- Respond to their concerns and preferences
- Share with patients, in a way they can understand, the information they want or need to know about their condition, its likely progression, and the treatment options available to them, including associated risks and uncertainties
- Respond to patients' questions and keep them informed about the progress of their care
- Make sure that patients are informed about how information is shared within teams and among those who will be providing their care
- Make sure, wherever practical, that arrangements are made to meet patients' language and communication needs.

Common questions

'How do you break bad news?' or *'A patient has metastatic colon cancer. How would you go about "breaking the bad news"?'*

The SPIKES approach, which can be applied to any situation, is a useful prompt for remembering the salient points when 'breaking bad news'.

Setting

- Ensure that you have all of the information beforehand and that you are adequately prepared
- Turn your bleep off and ensure there are no interruptions
- Ensure the room is quiet
- Ensure a member of nursing staff is also present.

Patient perception

- Determine what is already known.

Invitation to discuss/share bad news

- Forewarn the patient/family that you want to discuss a difficult topic
- Obtain permission to discuss or share the bad news.

Knowledge

- Gauge the level or amount of information the patient wants
- Give information appropriate to the patient's level of understanding/ background and avoid medical jargon
- Information should be sufficient for the patient to make an informed decision as to their management
- Repeatedly check that the patient has understood what you have told them.

Emotions

- Be empathetic, sensitive to the reactions you are likely to generate, warm, honest and to the point
- Leave time for questions to be asked.

Strategy and Summary

- Finally, summarize the salient points of the conversation
- Formulate a strategy/plan and give a realistic timeframe for this

- Check the patient's understanding of what they have been told
- Identify if the patient has any specific concerns
- Offer written additional material, e.g., information leaflets
- Offer the patient your contact details.

(See also the Empathy and sensitivity + communication skills section in Further reading.)

Associated questions

Questions such as the 'patient that refuses an operation' or the 'patient that refuses treatment and wishes to self-discharge' are common. Good communication (i.e., listening, negotiation and compromise to reach resolution) is usually the mainstay in management of these scenarios.

When dealing with 'difficult' patients it is important to exclude any organic pathology, such as sepsis or psychosis, which may be contributing to their behaviour.

In general, when dealing with 'difficult' patients you should:

- Be professional
- Conduct the conversation in private
- Ensure that you are not disturbed, e.g., transfer your bleep, as this may aggravate a potentially volatile situation
- Have a chaperone/witness – ideally a nurse or colleague
- Listen to the patient's ideas, concerns and expectations (ICE) – this is the first step towards achieving resolution. It may be that the patient has legitimate concerns or has misunderstood the situation
- Remain calm if the patient gets irate and allow them to vent their concerns and feelings
- Acknowledge the patient's feelings, e.g., 'I can see that you are upset.'
- Empathize
- Do not be afraid to apologize if that is appropriate, e.g., 'I am sorry that your operation has been cancelled, but we had an emergency case which took priority.'
- Negotiate a compromise, e.g., 'What I can do is speak to the consultant's secretary and I will call you with your new appointment date.' You may be able to give the patient a number of options and you should mutually agree upon a course of action. Importantly, do not promise anything that you cannot deliver on.
- Finally, at the end of the consultation
  - Invite questions
  - Summarize the key points

○ Offer further support, e.g., follow-up appointment, your contact details, information leaflets.

Note: If at any point you feel out of your depth, you should enlist more senior help.

Organization and planning

Common questions

- How do you effectively organize your day?
- What advice would you give your Foundation Year 1 doctor on their first day at work?
- You should be a self-starter. Give a recent example that demonstrates that you have initiative.

Professional integrity and respect for others

Common questions

'How do you explain to a patient that a postoperative complication has arisen?'

The GMC gives clear guidance within *Good Medical Practice* (GMC 2006b) regarding the management of adverse events at work: 'If a patient under your care has suffered harm or distress, you must act immediately to put matters right, if that is possible. You should offer an apology and explain fully and promptly to the patient what has happened, and the likely short-term and long-term effects. … Patients who complain about the care or treatment they have received have a right to expect a prompt, open, constructive and honest response including an explanation and, if appropriate, an apology. You must not allow a patient's complaint to affect adversely the care or treatment you provide or arrange.'

'How do you prevent medical errors?'

Each year 15,000 NHS patients die or are seriously injured as a result of clinical error – more deaths than attributed to lung cancer. In addition, medical negligence costs the NHS approximately £400 million each year.

In an anonymous survey of over 4000 doctors conducted by Doctors.net.uk:

- 82% of participants reported that they had seen a colleague make a mistake or give suboptimal care
- 15% claimed that this mistake had led either to death or disability.

When asked what action was taken:

- 10% reported that they had done nothing
- A third said that they had spoken to their colleague
- <10% had reported the error via established channels.

Furthermore, 80% of all doctors surveyed admitted that they themselves had also made errors; again less than 10% had reported them.

Mechanisms to prevent medical error include:

- Promotion of reporting of error, e.g., confidential and easily accessible reporting systems (also known as critical incidence reporting)
- Promoting safety – through education of patients and staff, e.g., patient safety leaflets
- Minimize human error in
  - Tasks, e.g., through development of checklists, protocols and computerization (such as drug dispensing units and computer-generated reminders)
  - Equipment design, e.g., through standardization of equipment throughout hospitals
  - Environment, with an emphasis on building a blame-free culture.

Note: Infection control is covered as a separate topic earlier in the chapter.

'What do you understand by the term "medical professionalism"?'

'Medical professionalism signifies a set of values, behaviours, and relationships that underpins the trust the public has in doctors.' (RCP 2005)

Associated question

- What would you do if a patient gave you £100 as a token of his appreciation for your hard work?

Learning and personal development

Questions that fall under this umbrella aim to establish your commitment and knowledge of the speciality to which you have applied. You should be able to demonstrate focus and direction in your career development to date as well as self-motivation. This may be evidenced by previous posts held, membership of the relevant learned societies (e.g., Rouleaux for vascular surgery, British Association of Urological Surgeons (BAUS) for urology), attendance at courses or meetings relevant to your speciality and a speciality-specific research/audit interest. You should attempt to highlight these features of your application.

Common questions

'What skills do you hope to achieve over the next year? How would you go about ensuring that you achieve this?'

This question aims to gauge your self-motivation and ability to drive your own learning. Ways to facilitate gaining skills/training include:

- Establishing and agreeing goals early with your consultant trainer/ programme director
- Attending courses
- Using simulators
- Identifying training opportunities
- Ensuring and rectifying early any clashes with training opportunities on the rota.

'How do you see your speciality changing in the future/next 5 years?'

This question is designed to assess your commitment to your speciality of interest and your awareness of recent developments and future challenges in this field. It may involve discussion of the following:

- Joint accreditation/training programmes, e.g., radiology and vascular surgery, due to the need for vascular surgeons to develop interventional radiological skills
- New technologies, e.g., robotics, laparoscopic/minimally invasive surgical techniques
- Changing population, e.g., increasing popularity of bariatric surgery
- Centralization of services, e.g., cardiac catheterization services, trauma.

'What makes a good doctor?'

This question needs careful preparation and should be specific to you but include those characteristics as outlined in the GMC's document *Good Medical Practice* (GMC 2006b) which states: 'A good doctor makes the care of their patients their first concern: they are competent, keep their knowledge and skills up to date, establish and maintain good relationships with patients and colleagues, are honest and trustworthy, and act with integrity.'

When answering this question, you should try to bring in aspects of your own personality, such as good communication skills, team-playing, managerial and organizational skills, professionalism and commitment, as well as personal attributes, such as an awareness of your own limitations and a commitment to continuing professional development; whilst importantly, also demonstrating a knowledge of the GMC's document.

'Walk me through your CV/portfolio.' or 'Tell me about yourself/ background.'

This is a gift of a question, which places the ball firmly in your court. However, it is also a very easy question to answer badly. Remember that you only have a limited amount of time, so a 2-minute preamble into your personal details, hobbies, etc. is a waste of time. Try to structure your answer, demonstrating focus in your career pathway to date, commitment to your speciality and drive. You should summarize your clinical experience and highlight your strengths and achievements and outline where you see yourself in the near future.

'What are your main strengths? What are your main weaknesses?'

These are common questions in interviews of all descriptions and need to be prepared properly beforehand. It is useful before the interview to review your CV and to make a list of your activities/achievements and against it list the skills which you have consequently developed. For example, secretary of the university rugby club – skills developed: teamwork, leadership and organization – and it is useful to bring these achievements into the discussion as evidence. Weaknesses are a more tricky area to broach. Reviewing any appraisals that you have had may be useful and provide some insight.

Leading on from these questions you may be asked, 'How do you handle stress?' This is an important question that is trying to assess how you behave under pressure.

'Why this deanery? Why should we give you the job here?'

You should have read the deanery website prior to the interview and you should have a good idea of how the training in the speciality that you are to be interviewed in is carried through within that particular deanery. You should also contact trainees already on the rotation to find out about the hospitals on the rotation and about any courses that they run locally or regionally which make training in that deanery better for you than elsewhere. If there are social reasons for applying, e.g., your partner works in that area, then now is your opportunity to state this. Discussing other interesting features of the region, e.g., facilities which may support a hobby, such as an excellent dry-ski slope, although not strictly related to medicine, are other ways of making the answer to this question more interesting.

'Why this speciality?'

You should prepare carefully for this question. Much of the answer should be related to your clinical experience of this speciality and, where possible, academic work that you have undertaken in this field. Try to make your answer interesting rather than just purely factual.

Associated questions

- Doctors need to be responsible for organizing their own learning and later, their clinical practice. Give an example where you have demonstrated this ability.
- Where do you see yourself in the medium and long term?
- What skills and attributes do you have which make you suitable for a higher career in this speciality?
- How have you demonstrated your commitment and aptitude for this speciality?
- What are your career intentions?
- What are the advantages or disadvantages of this speciality?
- Tell me about your most proud achievement.
- Tell me about your hobbies and how they have affected the way you practise medicine.
- What efforts (e.g., activities or achievements) have you made to increase your insight and capabilities relevant to this speciality?
- How have you demonstrated your commitment to this speciality?

References

British Medical Association. (2007) *Referral Management Principles*. BMA, London.

Cooksey D. (2006) *A Review of UK Health Research Funding*. HM Treasury, London. http://www.hm-treasury.gov.uk/media/4/A/pbr06_cooksey_final_report_636.pdf

Department of Health. (1997) *The New NHS: Modern, Dependable*. DH, London. http://www.archive.official-documents.co.uk/document/doh/newnhs/contents.htm

Department of Health. (1998) *A First Class Service: Quality in the New NHS*. DH, London.

Department of Health. (2000a) *The NHS Plan: A Plan for Investment, A Plan for Reform*. DH, London.

Department of Health. (2000b) *Improving Working Lives Standard: NHS Employers Committed to Improving the Working Lives of People Who Work*. DH, London.

Department of Health. (2002a) *Unfinished Business: Proposals for Reform of the Senior House Officer Grade*. A report by Sir Liam Donaldson, Chief Medical Officer for England. DH, London. http://www.mmc.nhs.uk/Docs/Unfinished-Business.pdf

Department of Health. (2002b) *Delivering 21st Century IT Support for the NHS: National Strategic Programme*. DH, London. http://www.dh.gov.uk/en/Publicationsandstatistics/Publications/PublicationsPolicyAndGuidance/DH_4008227

Department of Health. (2004a) *Modernising Medical Careers: The Next Steps – The Future Shape of Foundation, Specialist and General Practice Training Programmes*. DH, London.

Department of Health. (2004b) *National Standards, Local Action: Health and Social Care Standards and Planning Framework 2005/2006–2007/2008*. DH, London.

Department of Health. (2004c) *The NHS Improvement Plan: Putting People at the Heart of Public Service*. DH, London.

Department of Health. (2004d) *Agenda for Change*. DH, London.

Department of Health. (2005) *The Research Governance Framework for Health and Social Care*. 2E, DH, London.

Department of Health. (2006a) *Good Doctors, Safer Patients: Proposals to Strengthen the System to Assure and Improve the Performance of Doctors and to Protect the Safety of Patients*. DH, London.

Department of Health. (2006b) *Our Health, Our Care, Our Say*. DH, London.

General Medical Council. (2006a) *Guidance on Continuing Professional Development*. GMC, London. http://www.gmc-uk.org/education/continuing_professional_development/cpd_guidance.asp

General Medical Council. (2006b) *Good Medical Practice*. 4E, GMC, London.

HM Treasury. (2002) *The Wanless Report. Securing our Future Health: Taking a Long-term View*. HM Treasury, London. http://www.hm-treasury.gov.uk/Consultations_and_Legislation/wanless/consult_wanless_final.cfm

HPERU (Health Policy and Economic Research Unit). (2005) *Impact of Treatment Centres on the Local Health Economy in England*. BMA, London.

Kibbe DC, Kalunzy AD, McLaughlin CP. (1994) Integrating guidelines with continuous quality improvement: doing the right thing the right way to achieve the right goals. *Jt Comm J Qual Improv* **20**:181–91.

Lewis R, Hinton L. (2005) *Putting Health in Local Hands. Early Experiences of Homerton University Hospital NHS Foundation Trust*. King's Fund, London.

MMC Inquiry. (2008) *Aspiring to Excellence*. Final report of the independent inquiry into Modernising Medical Careers, led by Professor Sir John Tooke. MMC Inquiry, London. http://www.mmcinquiry.org.uk/MMC_FINAL_REPORT_REVD_4jan.pdf

Muir Gray JA. (1997) *Evidence-based Healthcare: How to Make Health Policy and Management Decisions*. Churchill Livingstone, London.

National Audit Office. (2002) *NHS Direct in England*. Report by the Comptroller & Auditor General. HC 505 Session 2001–2002. NAO, London.

NHS Executive. (1996) *Promoting Clinical Effectiveness: A Framework for Action in and through the NHS*. DH, London.

NHS Management Executive. (1999) *Introduction of Managed Clinical Networks in Scotland*. MEL(1999)10. NHS Management Executive. Edinburgh. http://www.show.scot.nhs.uk/publications/pubindex.htm

NHS Information Authority. (2003) *Data Standards: Responsible PCT*. NHS Information Standards Board. DSC Notice 19/2003. http://www.connectingforhealth.nhs.uk/dscn/dscn2003/192003.pdf

NHS Modernisation Agency. (2004) *Findings and Recommendations from the Hospital at Night Project.* NHS Modernisation Agency, London.

NICE & Healthcare Commission. (2002) *Principles of Best Practice in Clinical Audit.* Radcliffe Medical, Abingdon.

Postgraduate Medical Education and Training Board. (2005) *Workplace Based Assessment.* A paper from the PMETB Sub-committee on Workplace Based Assessment. PMETB, London.

Postgraduate Medical Education and Training Board. (2008) *A Trainee's Guide to the Postgraduate Medical Education and Training Board.* PMETB, London.

Roberts G. (2003) *Review of Research Assessment.* Report by Sir Gareth Roberts to the UK funding bodies. http://www.rareview.ac.uk/reports/roberts.asp

Royal College of Physicians. (2005) *Doctors in Society: Medical Professionalism in a Changing World.* RCP, London.

Sackett DL, Rosenberg WM, Gray JA, Haynes RB, Richardson WS. (1996) Evidence based medicine: what it is and what it isn't. *BMJ* **312**:71–2.

Smith R. (1992) Audit and research. *BMJ* **305**:905–6.

UK National Screening Committee. (2000) *What is Screening?* http://www.nsc.nhs.uk/whatscreening/whatscreen_ind.htm

Wilson JMG, Jungner G. (1968) *Principles and Practice of Screening for Disease.* Public Health Paper Number 34. WHO, Geneva.

Further reading

Audit

NHS Clinical Governance Support Team. (2005) *A Practical Handbook for Clinical Audit.* CGST, Leicester. http://www.cgsupport.nhs.uk/resources/Clinical_Audit/1@Introduction_and_Contents.asp

Wade DT. (2005) Ethics, audit and research: all shades of grey. *BMJ* **330**:468–71.

Clinical governance

Department of Health. (2001) *National Evidence-based Guidelines for Preventing Healthcare Associated Infections.* DH, London.

House of Commons Committee of Public Accounts. (2005) *Improving Patient Care by Reducing the Risk of Hospital Acquired Infections: A Progress Report.* House of Commons, London.

National Audit Office. (2000) *The Management and Control of Hospital Acquired Infections in Acute NHS Trusts.* NAO, London.

National Audit Office. (2004) *Improving Patient Care by Reducing the Risk of Hospital Acquired Infections: A Progress Report.* NAO, London.

Clinical knowledge and expertise

General Medical Council. (1998) *Seeking Patients' Consent: The Ethical Considerations.* GMC, London. http://www.gmc-uk.org/guidance/current/library/consent.asp

Empathy and sensitivity + communication skills

Baile WF, Buckman R, Lenzi R, et al. (2005) SPIKES – a six-step protocol for delivering bad news: application to the patient with cancer. *Oncologist* **5**:302–11.

Faulkner A. (1998) ABC of palliative care: communication with patients, families, and other professionals. *BMJ* **316**:130–2.

General Medical Council. (2006) *Good Medical Practice*. 4E, GMC, London.

Management

NICE. (2006) *About NICE Guidance: What Does It Mean for Me?* NICE, London. http://www.nice.org.uk/aboutnice/about_nice_guidance_what_does_it_mean_for_me.jsp

Other important areas within this section

Audit Commission. (2007) *Putting Commissioning into Practice*. Audit Commission, London.

King's Fund. (2007) *Practice-based Commissioning*. King's Fund, London.

Problem solving and decision-making

General Medical Council. (2002) *Withholding and Withdrawing Life Prolonging Treatments: Good Practice in Decision-making*. GMC, London.

Publications

Campbell M. (2002) *Statistics at Square One*. BMJ Books, London.

Harris M, Taylor G. (2003) *Medical Statistics Made Easy*. Martin Dunitz, London.

Research

GMC. (2002) *Research: The Role and Responsibilities of Doctors*. GMC, London. http://www.gmc-uk.org/guidance/current/library/research.asp

6 Difficult interview questions

Further interview questions, especially difficult or challenging interview questions will draw on multiple aspects of the person specification – for instance, those relating to conflict at work. This may be a conflict with a colleague, e.g., another junior doctor, a GP or a nurse; or it could be with a relative who may be questioning your management of a family member and they may be quite aggressive.

You need to formulate an example where this has occurred in your own practice and then answer how you dealt with it in terms of, first of all, your communication skills, and secondly, in terms of your team-working ability, as you may need to involve other members of the team, including your seniors. You must emphasize that you will listen to the views of all of those involved in the altercation and then negotiate some form of mutually acceptable resolution to the conflict.

Conflict-type questions are common and need careful preparation but the answer will inevitably involve communication skills, negotiation and initiative, empathy, team working and possibly also clinical incidence reporting.

Other common 'difficult' interview questions are those which deal with an underperforming colleague. Importantly, when answering these questions you should remember that you have a duty of care to your patient. *Good medical practice* clearly states, 'You must protect patients from risk of harm posed by another colleague's conduct, performance or health. The safety of patients must come first at all times. If you have concerns that a colleague may not be fit to practice, you must take appropriate steps without delay, so that the concerns are investigated and patients protected where necessary.'

Common questions

'How do you manage a colleague who is working under the influence of alcohol or drugs?'

In tackling this scenario, it is important to appreciate that a 'difficult' doctor may be a doctor in difficulty – i.e., they may be under work (conflict with colleagues/managers) or personal (domestic, financial, bereavement) pressure, ill, not coping (physically or mentally), insecure, inadequately trained, lack motivation, etc. – and additional stress at work (e.g., long commutes to and from work, shift-working, frustration at inefficiencies in the system, etc.) may be exacerbating matters.

There are a number of avenues available to you to resolve this matter:

- Local systems should be in place, and you should initially attempt to seek local resolution. If you feel you can, it may be appropriate to talk to the doctor involved directly. If not, you should contact an appropriate lead within your trust, e.g., clinical director, educational supervisor, senior clinician or deanery.
- If there is no one appropriate you can speak to, or if you feel the system in place has been ineffective, you should contact the GMC.

If you are unsure how to progress, you could discuss your concerns with an impartial colleague, your medical defence union, the BMA or the GMC.

If you decide to approach the colleague, in general:

- Be open, i.e., acknowledge there is a problem – don't simply just avoid or ignore, minimize it, as it could lead to a medical error
- Tackle the problem early – don't leave it to escalate
- Listen
- Focus any criticism on the behaviour, not the person; highlighting the person's strengths is a good way of engaging the person
- Avoid blame
- Avoid being confrontational and judgemental, or labelling the person
- Offer to negotiate differences but not compromise
- Be supportive in helping the person to accept their problem and to find practical solutions, e.g., job restructuring, retraining, educational support, counselling, mentoring
- Evaluate the possible solutions
- Decide together upon the best course of action and how to take it forward
- Monitor progress and be clear on your expected goal.

Alternatively, in some instances (not the above), you may want to take a team approach to tackling the situation, e.g., have a team discussion on the how the team is doing, without focusing on the 'difficult' member.

Associated questions

- 'How do you approach a colleague who is always late for work?'
- 'Your patient has suffered an acute myocardial infarction and is in heart failure. You have called the cardiology SpR and he is refusing to review the patient. How would you tackle the situation?'
- 'How would tackle a 'difficult' colleague?'
- 'Where can doctors go for help?'
- 'Two of your colleagues do not get along, and this is impacting on patient care. How would you resolve this conflict?'

'How would you tackle bullying/harassment in the workplace?'

> 'Bullying and harassment is unwanted conduct affecting the dignity of people in the workplace and may be related to age, sex, religion, race, disability, sexual orientation or any other personal characteristic. It may be persistent or an isolated event, but in all cases, the actions or comments are viewed as demeaning and unacceptable to the victim.' (BMA 2006)

Bullying and harassment is common within the NHS. In a survey of NHS staff in 2006 by NHS Employers, 8% reported that they had experienced bullying, (11% by colleagues), and less than 50% had reported it.

In general, bullying and harassment in the NHS may be tackled by:

- Operating a policy of zero tolerance within trusts and medical schools
- Raising awareness of bullying and harassment within trusts and medical schools
- Each NHS trust and deaneries developing and implementing a policy for dealing with bullying and harassment. This policy should:
  - Be publicized to new and existing staff
  - Have staff trained to deliver it
  - Require training of managers and those responsible for dealing with complaints of this nature
  - Include confidential support services for all parties affected, e.g., trained support workers, counselling, independent mediators, work in conjunction with the complainant's trade union.

In the first instance, resolution of the complaint is usually achieved through mediation via an informal procedure and a formal procedure in the event of failure of the former.

'A patient's family does not agree with your decision regarding a DNAR (Do not attempt resuscitation) order. How would you tackle this?'

Discussions around DNAR orders can be incredibly difficult and usually very distressing for both patients and those close to them. Despite this, where appropriate, you should always attempt to inform patients and involve them in the decision-making process. All cardiopulmonary resuscitation (CPR) decisions should be made on an individual basis and importantly, and relevant to this scenario, 'neither patients, nor those close to them, can demand treatment that is clinically inappropriate. If the healthcare team believes that CPR will not re-start the heart and breathing … it should not be offered or attempted.' (Resuscitation Council (UK) 2007)

This scenario requires you to demonstrate diplomacy and good communication. Prior to your discussion with the relatives, you should consult other members of the team from both primary and secondary care (e.g., GP, nurses) to gauge their views and during the consultation:

- Be sensitive
- Listen to the family and explore their ideas, concerns and expectations (ICE), regarding CPR – it may very well be that they have misunderstood or have unrealistic expectations of what CPR entails
- Provide realistic information, in terms of the patient's best interests, regarding:
  - What CPR involves, e.g., chest compressions, giving the heart electric shocks, use of drugs, ventilation
  - The likelihood of a successful outcome – for example, survival and morbidity (e.g., long-term disability due to brain damage, prolonged admission to ITU, long-term artificial ventilation)
  - Risks (e.g., sternal fractures, splenic/hepatic rupture) a traumatic and undignified death for the patient.
- Emphasize that a DNAR order pertains purely to CPR in the event of a cardiac or respiratory arrest and does not imply withdrawal or withholding of life-sustaining treatment, e.g., fluids, antibiotics, and physiotherapy
- Diplomatically inform relatives that they have no legal authority but do play an important role in informing the decision-making process
- Advise the family that should their relative's condition improve, the order would be re-evaluated
- Record the discussion and its outcome
- If a second opinion is requested, this should be given
- It may be appropriate if an agreement cannot be reached to:
  - Transfer the patient to the care of another team
  - Seek legal advice.

The responsibility for the DNAR decision ultimately lies with the most senior clinician; however, they may delegate this duty to another member of the team who is competent to make this decision. In this scenario, you may need to and should not be afraid to ask for more senior help.

Note: In cases where patients have capacity to make decisions regarding their health, you should seek their permission before sharing information with either family or friends.

In general, when discussing DNAR decisions with relatives it is recommended (Resuscitation Council (UK) 2007) that you should:

- Offer patients as much information as they want (or, if the patient lacks capacity, those close to them)
- Provide information in a manner and format which patients can understand; this may include patient information leaflets
- Provide an interpreter if necessary
- Answer questions as honestly as possible
- Explain the aims of treatment.

'Your consultant has a wound infection rate of 70%. What would you do?'

Patient safety is of prime importance in these types of question. In general, the approach is to:

- Document/log these 'critical' events, e.g., through critical incidence reporting, audit or your own records
- Formally raise your concerns early. Possible avenues include:
  - Your clinical director
  - Formal whistleblowing channels
  - The police, if you suspect a criminal offence has occurred.
- Speak to colleagues informally:
  - For confidential advice, e.g., your educational supervisor, the clinical director, your consultant
  - To investigate whether the problem has been experienced or observed by others
- Seek independent advice, e.g., from the GMC, BMA and Public Concern at Work (www.pcaw.co.uk)
- In addition, it may be appropriate for you to approach your consultant (as it is in this scenario) directly.

The Public Interest Disclosure Act (PIDA), also known as the 'whistleblower's law', came into force in 1999 and encourages people to raise concerns about malpractice in the work place whilst also protecting whistleblowers from any forms of reprisal, e.g., bullying. All trusts should have a well-publicized, formal 'whistleblowing' policy, which should:

- Contain details of named managers responsible for investigating staff concerns about malpractice
- Respect the anonymity and confidentiality of staff raising the concern
- Offer mechanisms to raise the concern outside the line management structure
- Advise regarding external routes through which the concern can be pursued, should internal routes fail.

Underperformance may be tackled via two key mechanisms:

- *Internally*, in conjunction with the National Clinical Assessment Authority, an organization that acts as a source or expertise, support and advice with assessment of the case and development and agreement of a remedial plan of action. This, however, requires cooperation from the doctor under investigation
- *Formally*, through referral to the GMC.

Associated questions

- 'A consultant you work for is managing a patient outside NICE guidelines. How do you approach this situation?' (see DH 2003, 2005)

'How do you deal with a complaint?'

The NHS complaints system essentially has three levels at which a complaint can be lodged and each should be attempted in a sequential fashion until an agreeable endpoint is achieved: These levels are:

1. Local resolution – i.e., through the Patient Advice Liaison Service (PALS), located within each NHS trust; complaints involving GPs are more difficult to resolve at this level.
2. Independent review through the Healthcare Commission.
3. Scrutiny of the complaint by the Health Service Ombudsman.

'What is the Patient Advice & Liaison Service (PALS)'

The Patient Advice & Liaison Service (PALS) was established following publication of *The NHS Plan* (DH 2000) and aims to: 'provide information, signposting to other services and help to resolve problems for patients, service users and carers. They act as a resource for staff and a source of intelligence for service improvement.' (DH 2006)

References

BMA. (2006) *Bullying and Harassment of Doctors in the Workplace*. BMA, London. http://www.bma.org.uk/ap.nsf/Content/bullying2006.

Department of Health. (2000) *The NHS Plan: A Plan for Investment, A Plan for Reform*. DH, London.

Department of Health. (2003) *Maintaining High Professional Standards in the Modern NHS: A Framework for the Initial Handling of Concerns about Doctors and Dentists in the NHS*. DH, London.

Department of Health. (2005) *Maintaining High Professional Standards in the Modern NHS: Directions on Disciplinary Procedures*. DH, London.

Department of Health. (2006) *Developing the Patient Advice & Liaison Service: Key Messages for NHS Organisations from the National Evaluation of PALS*. DH, London.

Resuscitation Council (UK). (2007) *Decisions Relating to Cardiopulmonary Resuscitation*. A joint statement from the British Medical Association, the Resuscitation Council (UK) and the Royal College of Nursing, London. http://www.resus.org.uk/pages/dnar.htm

Further reading

Department of Health. (2000) *The NHS plan: A Plan for Investment, A Plan for Reform*. DH, London.

Department of Health. (2006) *Good Doctors, Safer Patients: Proposals to Strengthen the System to Assure and Improve the Performance of Doctors and to Protect the Safety of Patients*. DH, London. http://www.dh.gov.uk/en/Publicationsandstatistics/Publications/PublicationsPolicyAndGuidance/DH_4137232

7

Other types of interview

Portfolio-based interviews

Some interviews may have a separate portfolio station, where questions, as the title of the station suggests, will be orientated around the candidate's portfolio. The objective of questioning here is to ensure that a candidate's portfolio is able to provide the supporting evidence to corroborate what the trainee has said in answer to a question. This evidence may be the interviewee's electronic logbook demonstrating the procedures performed or be in the form of recorded DOPs (directly observed procedures), mini-CEX (mini-clinical evaluation exercises), CBDs (case-based discussions) and PBAs (procedure-based assessments) which may be used to illustrate, for instance, commitment to the speciality.

Portfolios should include the following:

- Your curriculum vitae (CV)
- Exam certificates
- Certificates of course attendance
- Posters presented at learned meetings
- Presentations including at journal clubs
- Abstracts and papers (full texts)
- Audit projects (full texts)
- Your personal development plan or educational contract
- A statement of your personal values – i.e., a health and probity statement
- Record of in-training assessments (RITAs)
- Workplace based assessments (WPBAs)
  - 360-degree assessments or mini-peer assessment tools (mini-PATs)
  - DOPs
  - Mini-CEX

    ○ Case-based discussions
    ○ Procedure-based assessments
- Appraisals
- A reflective log of activities and experience
- Logbook of clinical e.g., procedures or operations activity or record of achieved competencies signed by your trainer
- References (usually structured).

Importantly, your portfolio should be kept in an orderly fashion and you must be familiar with all sections of it, as during the course of interview you may need to produce the relevant supporting documentary evidence, e.g., course or meeting attendance certificates as evidence of continuing professional development.

Common questions

'What have you learnt whilst putting together your portfolio?'

The key perceived learning advantages of developing a portfolio include:

- Encourages self-reflection with a positive impact on future practice and approach to problems
- Identifies personal strengths and weaknesses
- Facilitates self-directed learning and personal development
- Improves and develops communication skills.

The above should be discussed in the context of your portfolio, with relevant examples.

Associated questions

- 'Why do you think it is important to maintain a portfolio?'
- 'Talk me through your portfolio'
- 'What are your strengths/weaknesses as evidenced by your portfolio?'

Assessment of communication skills at interview

Importantly, your communication skills are likely to be continuously assessed throughout the course of the interview and it is therefore essential that you are continuously aware of your body language – the way you are sitting, listening to the interviewer, thinking through your responses to questions – and that you avoid monosyllabic responses.

If you are asked a direct question about how you rate your communication skills then you should be positive. Don't use single word answers such as 'average' or 'satisfactory' – use full sentences which demonstrate that you have good communication skills.

In addition, communication skills can be more formally assessed in a number of other ways at interview. You may be asked to give a presentation (this may or may not be pre-planned). Some interviews will merely assess the content of presentations but others will mark the context as well. Communication skills can also be assessed in a station with a trained actor/actress using defined scenarios.

Communication skills will score more highly in some specialties compared to others.

Assessment of practical skills at interview

An additional station may be present in some interviews, which is designed specifically to assess practical ability. This is more likely to be present in the craft specialties and will, generally speaking, involve quite simple tasks such as suturing and tying knots. Some skills may require familiarity with commonly used instruments in that speciality. For instance, in otolaryngology, familiarity with microscopes would be an important practical skill. Undoubtedly in the future, practical skills will play a much more important part in the interview process than they do currently.

Examples

- 'Assume I am a medical student attached to your firm. Teach me how to tie a knot/perform an interrupted stitch'
- 'Perform a cranial nerve examination.'

Assessing presentation skills at interview

Basically there are two ways in which presentations can be incorporated into the interview process.

First, you may be asked to attend the interview with a prepared talk on PowerPoint. Strict instructions are usually given as to the length of the talk and it is essential that you keep well within this time, as you may be cut short if you don't. This may result in you not being able to make some of your most important points. The topics chosen will vary speciality by speciality but nearly always tend to be generic, such as, 'Why have you chosen this speciality?' or 'What is your commitment to training in this speciality?' There should be plenty of time before the interview to prepare for this type of presentation and to make sure that you fully understand the subject matter. You should expect to be asked and be prepared to answer questions on your presentation and subject area, e.g., 'Why have you chosen this particular topic?'

In the second type of presentation you will be asked just prior to going into the interview to make a 2- or 3-minute presentation and you may or may not be allowed to use visual aids (if visual aids are allowed, this will usually be in the form of a single overhead transparency). In addition you may or may not be allowed to refer to your portfolio. Questions in this type of interview are likely to be generic, e.g., 'Why are you the best person for the job?' or 'Describe your strengths and weaknesses', and other examples include questions that have already been discussed in this chapter. The purpose of this second type of presentation, in addition to assessing your communication and presentation skills, is to assess your ability to think on your feet and to be dynamic.

General tips on preparing your presentation

- Your presentation should be in Microsoft PowerPoint and in landscape
- Your first slide should contain the presentation title and your name only
- Do not overcrowd your slides; ideally there should be no more than 4 or 5 bullet points or 9–15 words per slide
- As a rule of thumb, you should expect to take 30–40 seconds per slide (may be up to 2 minutes for more complex slides) and you should adjust the total number of slides to your time limit
- Choose the size of your font carefully – ideally it should be size 28 or greater
- Avoid using a busy or distracting background – i.e., stick to a plain or non-offensive slide background
- Choose your text and background colours carefully and try and avoid reds and greens as your interviewers may be colour blind
- Avoid excess animation and focus on the content of your presentation; now is not the time to work on getting laughs
- Don't simply read your slides – the bullets on the slides should merely be a prompt and summary of the salient points. Keep this simple
- Speak clearly and confidently, and make eye contact with the interviewers
- Pace the presentation – don't suddenly realize in the last 30 seconds that you still have a third of the presentation left to go through
- Practise your presentation and if possible do this in front of friends or

colleagues and get them to comment on ways that you could improve your presentation. Also, get them to ask you questions

- You *must* make sure that you keep to time
- When delivering your presentation, watch where you stand and ensure you don't obscure or detract attention from your slides
- If you are likely to need a laser pointer, take one of these along with you to the interview as one may not always be available
- Draw up a list of the possible questions that you may be asked in relation to the topic you are presenting on and be prepared to answer these
- When answering questions, don't be defensive or argumentative
- Bring a back-up copy of your presentation, e.g., on an additional memory-stick.

Where you are given only a short period of time to prepare a presentation, the same general principles as above can be applied.

Finally, remember the interviewers will expect you to be nervous, so don't worry if you stutter or the presentation doesn't go quite to plan.

8

After the interview

So you got the job …

Accepting the job

The highest ranked candidates will be given a job offer following completion of interviews for that speciality. Job offers will be made locally by individual deaneries, and you will be asked to decline or accept the offer within a set timeframe. The MMC Programme Board has agreed that applicants will have a minimum of 48 hours (excepting weekends and public holidays) to accept or decline the offer of a post. Following this period, posts which are left unfilled/declined can be re-offered to other candidates who are eligible, allowing deaneries to fill as many posts as possible. If posts still remain, these will be re-advertised for the next round of applications. Importantly, candidates can only accept one job offer and the offer for appointment is made under the condition that a post has not been accepted elsewhere.

Fixed term speciality training appointments (FTSTAs)

Fixed term speciality training appointments (FTSTAs) will be allocated at the same time as speciality training (ST3) places. However, if a candidate accepts an offer of an FTSTA, and at a later date (i.e. following the return of unfilled posts) is offered a specialty training post, they may accept the specialty training offer and decline the previously accepted FTSTA offer. This only applies to FTSTAs and you cannot inter-change between FTSTAs.

What next ...

The BMA provides clear advice to junior doctors (summarized below) on their website (www.bma.org.uk/ap.nsf/Content/acceptingoffers) regarding questions you should ask before accepting any job offer. Time between receiving and accepting the offer is tight, however, and although you may feel pressurized to accept the job, it is well worth ascertaining the following to avoid surprises further down the line:

- Your start date
- Your annual pay and incremental date
- Details regarding your first post on the rotation
  - Where you will start and department
  - Pay-banding of the post, e.g., 1A, 1B, 1C, 2A, 2B or 2C
- What the endpoint of training will be – i.e., CCT, generalist
- Future posts in the rotation and their pay-banding
- The removals and travel expenses policy within the deanery or at your employer and your eligibility to claim these expenses
- Accommodation available including on-call facilities and accommodation
- Type of rota you will work, e.g., shift pattern, frequency of shifts
- Annual and study leave entitlement and required notice, and whether locum cover will be provided.

If in doubt, BMA members should contact *ask*BMA.

Following the offer of a job and your acceptance to a training programme, the deanery will provide your future employer with the following information:

- Your application form and signed references, where available
- A copy of your medical school qualification certificate and other qualification certificates
- A copy of your passport details or recognized identity card
- A copy of your GMC certificate
- A job offer letter, details of your type of contract and your start date.

The NHS employer is responsible for conducting pre-employment checks, following which they will issue you with a formal letter of appointment and a contract of employment, which should comply with the nationally agreed terms and conditions of service for all junior doctors. Your NHS employer should contact you to inform you that the pre-employment checks are being conducted. In order to complete a pre-employment check, the following documents are required:

- Signed and validated professional references
- Health clearance by occupational health

- Criminal records – i.e., Criminal Records Bureau (CRB) clearance
- GMC registration
- Evidence of the right to work in the UK
- Verification of your identity.

It is important to note that a contract of employment cannot be issued if there is any documentation (e.g. references) outstanding and it is your responsibility to ensure that your human resources/medical personnel department receive these.

Job inductions

The first trust that you are employed to on your rotation is responsible for providing a detailed induction, which is both trust and specialty specific. This should be arranged in conjunction with the postgraduate centre within each trust and trust human resources and occupational health departments and your educational/clinical supervisor.

So you didn't get the job ...

Requesting feedback

All interview candidates will be able to obtain feedback regarding their performance from the deanery. In the first instance, this is usually just your ranking following the short-listing and interview process; however, you should contact the relevant deanery and request more in-depth feedback as well as careers advice. All deaneries should have a designated careers advisor. In addition, advice can be sought from a number of other sources, namely:

- Your current educational supervisor
- Careers advisors within the Royal Colleges
- BMA Careers Service.

What now ...

It essential that you reflect on all aspects of the interview process – from your application to your portfolio – as well as your actual performance in the interview. It may be that there are very obvious 'areas of weakness' in either your application form or interview technique. Often, however, these weaknesses are far more subtle.

Having identified the areas for improvement, the key question is whether they can be realistically improved upon in the timeframe that you have until your next application. If the answer is no, you will need to think hard and make the tough decision of whether or not you would in fact be better off cutting your losses and applying to a different specialty.

These are difficult assessments and choices to make and not ones that you should undertake without seeking support or advice from the relevant organizations or people.

INDEX